HEALTHCARE REFORM
IN AMERICA

A Reference Handbook

Other Titles in ABC-CLIO's
**Contemporary
World Issues**
Series

Books in the Contemporary World Issues series address vital issues in today's society such as genetic engineering, pollution, and biodiversity. Written by professional writers, scholars, and nonacademic experts, these books are authoritative, clearly written, up-to-date, and objective. They provide a good starting point for research by high school and college students, scholars, and general readers as well as by legislators, businesspeople, activists, and others.

Each book, carefully organized and easy to use, contains an overview of the subject, a detailed chronology, biographical sketches, facts and data and/or documents and other primary-source material, a directory of organizations and agencies, annotated lists of print and nonprint resources, and an index.

Readers of books in the Contemporary World Issues series will find the information they need in order to have a better understanding of the social, political, environmental, and economic issues facing the world today.

HEALTHCARE REFORM
IN AMERICA

A Reference Handbook

Jennie Jacobs Kronenfeld
and Michael R. Kronenfeld

**CONTEMPORARY
WORLD ISSUES**

ABC-CLIO

Santa Barbara, California   Denver, Colorado   Oxford, England

Library of Congress Cataloging-in-Publication Data
Kronenfeld, Jennie Jacobs and Michael R. Kronenfeld
   Healthcare reform in America : a reference handbook / Jennie Jacobs Kronenfeld and Michael R. Kronenfeld
       p.   cm. — (Contemporary world issues)
   Includes bibliographical references and index.
   ISBN 1-57607-977-5 (hardcover : alk. paper); 1-57607-978-3 (eBook)
   1. Health care reform—United States—Handbooks, manuals, etc.
I. Kronenfeld, Michael R.   II. Title.   III. Series.

RA395.A3K7593   2004
362.1'0973—dc22

                                                                      2004005417

08   07   06   05   04   10   9   8   7   6   5   4   3   2   1

This book is also available on the World Wide Web as an eBook. Visit abc-clio.com for details.

ABC-CLIO, Inc.
130 Cremona Drive, P.O. Box 1911
Santa Barbara, California 93116-1911

This book is printed on acid-free paper ∞.
Manufactured in the United States of America.

Contents

Preface

In the last 100 years in the United States, the emergence of a national health system, such has been developed by almost every other developed country during this time period, has always seemed to be at least 5 to 10 years in the future. In the beginning of the twenty-first century, the problem is again becoming critical. Although some limited reforms have occurred in the 1990s (some control of managed care; CHIP program), many major problems remain, including those of limited access to care, concerns about quality, and issues about costs of care, rising costs of care, costs of health insurance, costs of prescription medicine, and consumer satisfaction. This handbook reviews the failed attempts of the last century, identifying the economic, social, and political issues that both pushed for the creation of a national system and prevented it from being implemented. These issues will then be reviewed in the context of today, the first decade of the twenty-first century, as healthcare reform issues will again be in the forefront of the political process.

Some of the key issues to be presented are:

- Cost of healthcare
- Access to healthcare
- The political process and healthcare reform

This handbook on healthcare reform presents issues and questions relevant to the full range of social science disciplines in high school and college level courses. By showing the interplay and significance of these issues as they focus on the healthcare system, the reader should be able to see the importance and interplay of the work of the different disciplines as they relate to concerns about healthcare delivery, healthcare reform, and healthcare policy.

This book is very different than it would have been if it had been written ten years ago before the emergence of the World Wide Web and the Internet as increasingly important platforms for the presentation of information, analysis, and advocacy on the relevant (and sometimes not so relevant) issues of our time. Before the Web, access to information and viewpoints on a topic were both limited and often untimely. Although many of the issue advocacy groups existed before the Web, finding out about them and obtaining information on them was both difficult and time consuming. Government data were available at many public and academic libraries but it was harder to find and access the relevant information. Periodical indexes were also available at libraries but they were harder to use and the tracking down of the articles identified was much more difficult and time consuming. Although the issues relating to the healthcare sector and the delivery of healthcare in the United States have not changed so greatly in this time period, the ability to access information on the topic has grown almost exponentially.

The ability to access large volumes of information about health and healthcare delivery, the healthcare sector more generally, and government programs relating to the delivery of healthcare has not necessarily made the task of understanding the issues any easier for someone just beginning to explore and understand them. It is very easy to become overwhelmed by the total volume of information now available. In addition to being overwhelmed by the volume, a more important and difficult issue is to assess the accuracy, utility, and perspective of the information presented by competing and contradictory advocacy groups. The first two chapters of this book should introduce the reader to the basic issues involved in healthcare reform and give the reader the context to use in the further exploration of the various issues relating to healthcare delivery and healthcare reform. As with learning about any new topic or using information presented by any individual or group advocating a specific viewpoint, a reader must be a careful "consumer" of the information presented on this topic that so directly impacts all of us.

We would like to thank many people for assistance in writing this book. Jennie's department chair, Verna Keith, and her associate chair, Deborah Sullivan, were helpful throughout the process, from, as good department administrators do, helping to facilitate time commitments to writing on certain days. Michael wants to thank Ted Wendel, associate provost for the Mesa Campus of ATSU, for his support and encouragement. He also wants to thank various advocacy groups who generously allowed us to reprint materials from their Web sites. If this book had been written five years earlier it would have been very different with an emphasis on print rather than Web-based sources. The World Wide Web provides a platform for the presentation of information, analysis, and advocacy on the various issues we face today. There is not a topic in which this is more evident than in the debate on the organization and reorganization of our healthcare sector with its direct impact on the health of us all.

Acknowledgments

We would also like to thank our family, our three sons, two of whom, Shaun and Aaron, were living at home while we were writing this book, Shaun in college and Aaron in his last two years of high school. Our third son, Jeffrey, was in his first and second years of college during this time. They were patient at times as we needed to work on aspects of the manuscript at home, helpful at times when we were discussing issues of healthcare reform by participating in discussions, and helping us to realize what the public more generally is and is not familiar with in terms of healthcare reform issues, and distracting at times as we had to deal with the life crises and concerns of teenagers and young adults in today's world.

1

Healthcare Reform: Cost, Quality, Access, and the Government's Role

Healthcare reform, or modification of the U.S. healthcare system so that affordable, high-quality healthcare services are available to everyone, is a public-policy issue that has received discussion in the United States off and on since World War II. The amount of discussion at any one time varies with changes in leading politicians and how much healthcare issues, including healthcare reform, are viewed as issues of high public concern. Just to look back at the most recent decades, the prominence of the topic of healthcare reform varied even between the two administrations of a single president; healthcare reform went from being a central issue in the first term of the Clinton administration to a position of lower concern by Clinton's second term. With the administration of George W. Bush, especially once the events of September 11, 2001, and the war with Iraq in 2003 led to a greater focus on international concerns and terrorism, the prominence of healthcare issues became fairly low. However, concerns about healthcare problems and the need for reform have not disappeared. For example, the need for Medicare reform and help for senior citizens in dealing with healthcare costs, especially drug costs, has again received discussion as the reality of election years approaches. Other issues will also revive attention to healthcare reform, since all of the major issues that led to the most recent failed attempt to pass major U.S. health reform legislation during the Clinton administration remain unresolved.

Why is there discussion about healthcare reform in the United States now? One reason is that, compared to almost all other industrialized countries in the world today, the United States has not resolved some very basic issues about the role of the government in the provision of care and in assuring that all citizens are able to receive good-quality care when they need it. In most of the world's industrialized countries, the government has been part of a process that guarantees access to many if not most healthcare services for all citizens. Not all countries arrive at the same solution for guaranteeing access for all. Some create a major national healthcare system (for example, Great Britain); others use more of a health insurance–based system. These insurance-based systems can vary widely. In Canada, there is a single-payer national health insurance system that some believe could be a model for reform in the United States. Unlike Great Britain, the system varies from one province to another (provinces are more or less the equivalent of states), and most physicians are still paid by health insurance, rather than on a yearly or per-patient salary. In Germany, nongovernmental insurance providers form the basis of the system, but there are various mechanisms in place to assure that all Germans are covered for most services. Many argue the United States does not really have a clear healthcare system but rather a confusing variety of public and private healthcare insurers and providers who function in different, and often competing, ways. Thus, while most countries have mechanisms in place to assure at least basic access to healthcare for all and to maintain quality while keeping overall costs reasonable, this is not true of the United States.

For almost fifty years, cost, quality, and access have been the three key watchwords for scholars in many of the different disciplines that study healthcare and the delivery of healthcare services. The name given to these types of studies and studies related to many aspects of the healthcare system is *health services research*. This name came into use about thirty years ago to describe research related to the use of, the organization and delivery of, the financing of, and the outcomes of health services such as quality of care and health status changes. Over the last fifteen years, it has become the most widely accepted term to describe interdisciplinary research on health and healthcare services. Disciplines that are often part of health services research include sociology, economics, political science, management sciences, epidemiology, and more applied fields such as public health, health services administration, health education, and policy sciences.

The importance of these three concepts (cost, quality, and access) should not be surprising, and, actually, these concepts are of primary importance with regard to many kinds of services that a person might receive, not just healthcare. For any service (or product), one thing of importance is the cost. For an individual about to visit a doctor (or a store), the simple question is, what must I pay? The more complicated question is whether the price is fair, reasonable, and appropriate. When this question is applied beyond the individual to a large group or the nation as a whole, we begin to ask questions such as, what are the total dollars being spent? how do these dollars relate to other kinds of services? and how do they relate to how much people in other places pay for these kinds of services?

A related question is, can I get the service or product? This is the concept of access. Access has at least two components—one component is simply the availability of the service. Are there doctors or hospitals around? Are the doctors taking new patients? Do the hospitals have empty beds? In healthcare, this question is often termed *geographical access* and is linked to specific places. Although the answers to policy questions about geographical access can be complex, the more complex side of access is *financial access,* or, do I have the money to pay for care? Increasingly in the United States, the answer to this question relates less to the amount of money any individual has in his or her wallet or bank account, and more to whether the person (and the person's family) has health insurance. The most important factor in having health insurance in the United States today is having a good job with benefits. In addition, certain categories of people, such as the elderly, many of the poor, and increasingly the children of the near poor, now have access to governmentally sponsored health insurance. Thus, access for an individual is partially linked to cost of care and also to specific aspects of that person's situation in the society. It is easy to see how access issues quickly become one major issue in healthcare reform.

Moving beyond the individual to the society as a whole, cost of care is linked to access, and at a broader policy level, this is particularly true. If a governmental unit, such as a state, is willing or able to spend a certain amount of dollars on healthcare for the poor and those without insurance, the state can provide more access to care to greater numbers of people if the average cost of care per person is $500 versus $1,000. Thus, as a public policy issue, costs and access are important and interrelated.

The third related concept is quality of care. Again, quality is a question we would ask about any type of service or even a specific product to be purchased. Is it a quality product, or is the care I will receive of high quality? Is it at least of acceptable quality? For consumer products, we often trade off between quality and cost. People decide to accept a less-well-made product (one that may not last as long—for example, disposable razors) if the price is lower. Once we begin to talk about a service such as healthcare, which involves the person's body and possibly entails life-or-death consequences, the willingness of many people to accept trade-offs between cost and quality is often low. Many people adopt the attitude that only the best quality is acceptable. In healthcare, experts discuss how everyone feels they deserve the best and most advanced care, even if they would not make the same choice about other goods and services. But what is the best quality? Are we always able to measure quality in healthcare? Consider an analogy to other service areas in American society. Although even the wealthiest people often eat fast food at some times and dine in elegant restaurants at other times, most people want elegant, outstanding healthcare at all times, not "fast food" healthcare. Issues of quality are very important and quickly become interwoven with policies about cost and access. That the government and individuals should not pay for inferior quality healthcare is a statement about which almost everyone agrees. But must everyone have the most technologically sophisticated care for it to be of high quality? The terms *two-tiered* and *two-class* were often used in the past to describe the U.S. healthcare system, with one tier or class for individually (and insured) paying patients and another for charity (or more recently, governmentally funded) patients. Providing different levels of quality of care is generally no longer viewed as appropriate, unless all of it is at a minimum standard of quality. Clearly, quality becomes a third major consideration, along with cost and access. The rest of this chapter will return to these and other related concepts, such as rising costs of healthcare and managed care, after a discussion of health policy formulation, the role of government, and a few comments about why healthcare reform has been harder to achieve in the United States than in many other countries in the world. Chapter 2 will focus on a review of healthcare reform efforts in the United States, looking more critically at the specifics of previous attempts at healthcare reform and also reviewing the development of the role of the federal government in healthcare. That chapter will focus on how healthcare issues have become government issues in the United States and on what has happened over the past one hundred years that left the United States in the position of being one of the only developed, industrialized countries that does not guarantee access to healthcare at some level to all of its citizens.

Health Policy Formulation and the Role of Government in Healthcare Reform

Healthcare reform is one part of U.S. health policy that has occupied an important place in the country's domestic policy agenda, and its importance within that agenda has been growing during the last thirty-five years. A nation's health policy is part of its overall social policy. Given that, health policy formulation is influenced by the variety of social and economic factors that impact social policy development. Generally, policies are authoritative decisions made in the legislative, executive, or judicial branch of government that are intended to influence the actions, behaviors, or decisions of others. If a policy relates to improvement of health, having enough healthcare professionals, or issues such as cost, quality, and access of healthcare services, it is a part of healthcare policy. In the United States today, the government plays a major role in the planning, directing, and financing of healthcare services, although this was less true in earlier time periods (Kronenfeld 1997).

Compared to some countries in the world, the United States has a complicated system of government that makes policy formulation and passage of subsequent enabling legislation difficult, not only in health but in other policy areas as well. The United States has a federal system of government, created by the U.S. Constitution. At the time of the founding of the country in the 1790s, federalism was a legal concept that defined the constitutional division of authority between the federal government and the states. Federalism stressed the independence of each level of government from the other while also incorporating certain functions (especially foreign policy) that were the exclusive area of the central (federal) government. Other policy areas, including healthcare, were initially conceived of as the states' responsibility. As a result of the expansion in domestic programs that began with the New Deal programs in the 1930s, an expanded role for the federal government in many areas has become an accepted aspect of the way government works in the United States today. Nonetheless, the complexity of a federal system still creates some complications in how health programs operate. Certain health programs are joint federal-state efforts. One of the biggest and best-known examples of such a joint effort in the health area is the Medicaid program, the program that provides healthcare coverage for many poor, lower-income Americans. Because this is a shared program in which both federal and state funds are used, but for which states must meet certain federal government rules, differences can occur between the two units of government. A cutback or an increase in mandated eligibility at the federal level may force a state to adjust its budget (Lee and Benjamin 1999). Meeting the state share of the program can be difficult for states in times of declining state revenues, such as during the recession in the United States that followed the September 11, 2001, terrorist attacks. In fact, the continued economic recession in the first half of 2003 has even led to some discussion in state legislatures about whether certain states will be able to provide the needed funds to continue to participate in Medicaid. During the last few decades, as eligibility for Medicaid has been expanded at certain points, states have had to find the dollars in their budgets to match the federal expenditures. These Medicaid match dollars have become one of the more rapidly rising areas of expenditure for states in recent decades. These complexities have become one cause behind the push from states for the federal government to become a major player in and leader of healthcare reform efforts.

In addition to the complexity the federal system creates across levels of government, government in the United States has other limitations. The U.S. Constitution contains notions of limited government resulting from the framers' fears of a strong central government and the importance they placed on protecting rights of individuals. Two important aspects that relate to these fears are the reserve clause and the creation of three branches of government. The reserve clause states that any powers not explicitly given to the federal government are reserved for the states, and this clause is the basis of the important role of states within the United States.

There are three branches of government in the United States: the executive, legislative, and judicial. At least in theory, these branches are separate and equal in power. Although popular culture in the United States has now exalted the executive branch, in the person of the president, to seem to be more powerful than the other branches, in reality the U.S. president is much less powerful than the heads of state under certain other political systems. In opposition to a parliamentary system of government like Great Britain's where the head of the party in the parliament is the prime minister, the head of the executive branch in the United States (the president) is separately elected from the legislative branch (Congress), and different political parties can be represented by the different branches. Thus, at any point in time, it may be much more difficult for the president's suggested policies to be enacted into law, since the president may represent a different political party than the party that controls Congress. This can be made even more difficult by there being two different legislative bodies represented with the Congress: the House of Representatives and the Senate. At any given time, the majority party of each branch of Congress can be different from the other branch; for example, the Senate may have a Republican majority while the House has a Democratic majority, or vice versa. In combination, this division of powers between units of government and between branches of government creates an institutional structure that makes reform policies and major policy changes more difficult to enact into laws. Under a parliamentary system, the prime minister can propose new policies and generally have those enacted into legislation, since the prime minister's party also controls the legislative branch of government. Generally, this has been given as one (although not the only) explanation of why major reforms, including reforms in the healthcare delivery system, are so difficult to accomplish in the United States (Steinmo and Watts 1995).

In addition, the presence of two different legislative bodies, the House of Representatives and the Senate, only compounds the difficulty of having healthcare reform legislation enacted. This is not accidental. The creation of two legislative bodies was part of a compromise between large and small states at the time of the writing of the Constitution. The House of Representatives was viewed as the body that was closer to the people, and each representative is responsible to and for a small district. Districts in each state are created in proportion to the percentage of the population in the United States that resides within that district, so that large or densely populated states have many more representatives in the House than do small or sparsely populated states. In contrast, each state has only two senators (no matter what the state's population), and they represent the entire state. Until the twentieth century, senators were not popularly elected but were appointed by the legislatures of the states. The two houses of Congress create a further opportunity for divided and weakened government, so that even if the party of the president wins a majority in one of the houses of the legislature, it still might not have a majority in both, thus making it more difficult for new ideas to be passed into law.

All of these structural factors in the basic operation of the government of the United States make it more difficult to have major policy changes enacted. Despite this, the role of the federal government in healthcare has expanded over the past several hundred years, and there have been times when change has occurred and other times when change appeared likely, yet failed politically. These specifics are discussed in Chapter 2.

Three Watchwords of the Healthcare System: Cost, Quality, and Access

Cost, quality, and access have been the three major watchwords of the healthcare system. What are the current trends in terms of those issues now? How do these three aspects of healthcare relate to each other? This section will review some basic patterns in each of these areas and then conclude by discussing some of the interactions between the three aspects.

Patterns of Health Insurance and Access to Care

Although there is a range of estimates about the numbers of people uninsured and underinsured in the United States from the early 1980s on, most sources agree that there has been an increase in the numbers of uninsured persons since the late 1970s (Wilensky and Ladenheim 1987; Freeman et al. 1987; Robert Wood Johnson Foundation 1987). Traditionally, the United States has always had many uninsured individuals. In fact, health insurance was not common in the United States prior to World War II, although some specialized groups did have insurance for some needs. During the 1950s, Blue Cross and Blue Shield plans began to operate in most states, and most municipal and state workers, as well as school employees, were given some form of coverage. Unionized employees increasingly also won health insurance coverage as a benefit. By the 1960s, coverage rates grew for people in many jobs and evolved into a typical benefit in many full-time jobs, including office, manufacturing, and government jobs. Some groups were less likely to be covered, especially those in service and retail jobs, the self-employed, and farm laborers.

By the early 1960s, most full-time workers and their families had some coverage, but if workers lost their jobs or retired, they and their families lost this coverage. Those without jobs, of course, generally did not have health insurance. Therefore, prior to the Medicaid program, income was a major determinant of access to care, especially access to outpatient and physician services. Because hospital care is typically for more urgent problems, people of more limited means often obtained hospital care in an emergency, sometimes as part of charity care provisions of hospitals. One of the policy successes of the 1960s was the passage of Medicare and Medicaid, which provided health insurance coverage to the elderly and the poorest who received welfare services. Over the next decades, Medicare also expanded to cover the disabled, the blind, and in 1972 persons with end-stage renal disease (ESRD) were added. Although at the time some people felt that Medicare would continue to expand and add additional disease categories and perhaps become the model for more comprehensive health insurance provided through the government, that has not happened. No new disease categories have been added to Medicare coverage since the addition of kidney diseases. Nonetheless, Medicare and Medicaid have increased the availability of healthcare services to the poor. Several studies have demonstrated that the gap in levels of physician use between the poor and the rest of society narrowed in the ten- to fifteen-year period after the passage of these programs (Wilson and White 1977; Aday, Anderson, and Fleming 1980).

In the late 1970s, the best estimates were that 25 to 26 million people in the United States were without healthcare insurance. This was about 13 percent of the population under age 65.

The numbers of uninsured grew in the 1980s. Estimates range from a low of 22 million to a high of 37 million uninsured persons (Robert Wood Johnson Foundation 1987; Wilensky and Ladenheim 1987; Wilensky 1987; Moyer 1989). From 1980 to the beginning of the new century, most sources agree that there has been an increase in the number of uninsured, with typical figures showing around 14 percent of people under 65 years of age with no coverage in 1984, up to 16 percent in 1996 and 17.4 percent in 1997, with small declines in 1998 and 1999, down to 16.6 and 16.1 percent respectively (Budrys 2001; Eberhardt, Ingram, and Makuc 2001). One clear pattern has been a decline in the percentage of people with private insurance coverage, such as through their workplace. For example, this figure declined from almost 77 percent in 1984 to 71 percent in 1996, and the percent uninsured would be higher except for a growth in Medicaid coverage in that same time frame, so that while only 7 percent of people under 65 had Medicaid coverage in 1984, almost 12 percent did in 1996, and the further expansions with the Children's Health Insurance Program (CHIP) program should continue to increase the percentage of children with government-based health coverage. In the United States today, most elderly persons are eligible for and are enrolled in Medicare, so that health insurance coverage rates in this group are very high. Recent immigrants are the group within the elderly least likely to have Medicare coverage.

Who are the Americans who have neither private health insurance nor coverage for healthcare services under public insurance programs such as Medicare and Medicaid? Why is this so important? One reason having some type of health insurance is so important is that health insurance coverage is an important determinant of access to care. When we discuss the uninsured, we are discussing those groups that are most likely to have major problems obtaining access to healthcare services. In general, about two in five American adults who do not have health insurance end up going without needed care (Cassil 1997). Uninsured adults are not a homogeneous group. Although some of the people without health insurance are those who we might assume are the major groups who would make up this population—the homeless, the socially dislocated—others are people who work in jobs either part or all of the year but nonetheless have no health insurance coverage, or those who are temporarily unemployed. Surprising to some people, those without insurance even include some relatively high-income families in which the primary breadwinner has a serious chronic illness, can no longer work, and yet is not a recipient of public health insurance programs.

Critical to understanding how some groups of people have no health insurance in American society today is the realization that most private health insurance in the United States is purchased through employer-based group insurance policies. These policies represent about 85 percent of all private coverage. By the late 1990s, rates of workplace health insurance coverage were lower than in the 1970s. One report in 1998 indicated that despite the nation's strong economy in the 1990s, the number of uninsured Americans continued an upward trend and was partially linked to size of employer. Although two-thirds of all workers in large firms of over 1,000 employees had health insurance, the figure declined to 52 percent in firms of 25 to 99 employees, and to less than 30 percent in firms of fewer than 25 employees (Aston 1998). Shifts in the sector of employment and shifts in the number of part-time versus full-time jobs are both related to ongoing changes in the economy. Many experts believe the United States has moved from a manufacturing-dominated economy to a service economy. Thus, typical changes would be decreases in the numbers of people employed in automobile manufacturing (a group with extensive health insurance coverage) and increases in the number of people employed in fast-food establishments. Many of these service-job employers pay only the minimum wage and often hire a large group of part-time workers. Typically, these part-time workers do not receive benefits such as health insurance. If the part-time worker is a high-school student covered under his or her parents' insurance or a person over sixty-five supplementing his or her Social Security income, the lack of health insurance provision in these jobs does not lead to an increase in the number of uninsured Americans. If these jobs are filled by heads of households or single adults who cannot obtain other jobs, however, there is an impact on the numbers of persons without health insurance.

In a more recent study of why workers are uninsured, special survey data were used to try to understand more about linkages between employment and health insurance status (Thorpe and Florence 1999). The 1997 Current Population Survey (CPS) data were combined with data from a special survey of workers including workers in contingent jobs (that is, those designed to last a specified period of time) and workers who are independent contractors or workers for temporary agencies. These types of work settings have been growing over the last decade. About 72 percent of all workers in this study were employed by a firm that offered health insurance coverage. Of these workers, 11 percent were not eligible for the coverage typically because of the number of hours worked. Some people do not actually enroll in the coverage offered by an employer. About 85 percent of eligible workers accepted coverage. About two-thirds of those who turned down coverage did so because they were covered by another family member, and some had purchased their own private insurance. About 22 percent of workers who declined coverage were uninsured. The high cost of insurance was generally cited as the most important factor in the decision to decline coverage. Of the ineligible workers, 37 percent were uninsured, 11 percent received some form of public coverage already, and 44 percent were insured through another family member. The survey also included information on workers in firms that did not offer any health insurance coverage. Of those, 40 percent were uninsured. Several suggestions are provided by the authors of this study. They recommend that, absent comprehensive healthcare reform, some smaller reforms could be helpful. Workers in alternative-type jobs, at all income levels, are less likely to be eligible for employee health insurance plans and more likely to be uninsured. It would be possible to increase the eligibility of such workers for benefits. Similarly, nondiscrimination workplace rules could be modified to include those working less than 20 hours per week. Such changes would probably make 3.5 million more workers eligible for health insurance (Thorpe and Florence 1999). Whether those workers would be able to afford such insurance remains an issue.

Some of the people without health insurance coverage are people with special health problems, especially those with a history of serious medical problems. Many people with serious health problems do maintain health insurance coverage as long as they keep their jobs. If they lose their current jobs due to the general economy or their health but can still work, they may experience problems in finding employment because of their health. Not only do businesses not want employees with illnesses that may require repeated absences, but, increasingly, health insurance companies are "experience rating" individual company policies. A workplace with a few high utilizers of healthcare due to chronic illness can raise the insurance rates for the entire company. Employers are thus more reluctant to hire a worker who may increase overall costs in this area. Although people who are medically uninsurable are a small part of those without health insurance, they represent a much larger proportion of the uncompensated care expenses because they are very high utilizers of health services.

Some other social factors are also important in the lack of health insurance coverage. Nationally, the age-adjusted percentage of the nonelderly population without health insurance varies by urbanization levels. Residents of fringe counties of metropolitan areas are least likely to lack coverage, while residents of central cities and nonmetropolitan counties are most likely to lack coverage (Eberhardt, Ingram, and Makuc 2001). Race or ethnicity also matters. In fact, Hispanics are the group least likely to have health insurance coverage, and this has been true for almost two decades. In 1984, about 29 percent of all Hispanics did not have any health insurance, as compared with 12 percent of white non-Hispanics and 20 percent of African American non-Hispanics. Ten years later, in 1994, the lack of health insurance had increased slightly for Hispanics and white non-Hispanics (32 and 14 percent, respectively) and had not really changed for African Americans. In 1998 and 1999, Hispanics remained the group with the highest percentage of its population lacking health insurance (about 34 percent versus figures of 14 to 12 percent for whites and 19 to 21 percent for African Americans). Within the Hispanic population, it is people of Mexican origin who are the most likely to lack health insurance. About 35 percent of Mexican-origin Hispanics lacked health insurance in 1984, and this increased to 38 percent by 1999 (Eberhardt, Ingram, and Makuc 2001).

The newest concern about potentially growing rates of the uninsured relates to the economy. With the economy slowing down and workers being laid off, fewer people may have access to employer-provided coverage. The unemployment rate grew from 4 percent in December 2000 to 5.4 percent in October 2001, following the terrorist attacks of September 11 (Rising Unemployment 2001). Since then, the economy has shown great volatility, especially in terms of stock market values. In addition, confidence levels in business have decreased, in part as a result of business ethics scandals, such as the Enron debacle. One recent estimate was that 75 million Americans, or 30.1 percent of the population, were uninsured at some point during 2001 or 2002. Ninety percent of these people were uninsured for at least three months, and about 80 percent were in working families (Meckler 2003).

Not only are rates of unemployment increasing, leading to higher percentages of people without health insurance, but the costs of premiums for health insurance are also increasing, at fairly rapid rates. Premiums for employer-provided health insurance grew 11 percent in 2001, the largest increase in a decade. Although the federal COBRA legislation now allows people laid off from firms with 20 or more employees to continue their healthcare coverage at group rates, workers must pay the entire premium once laid off. This payment is often much higher than when they were employed since many employers subsidize the cost of health insurance for their employees. The average employer-sponsored coverage now without employer subsidy is $2,650 for the employee and over $7,000 for family coverage. For many unemployed workers, this amount is prohibitive. A recent analysis argues that for every 100 persons who lose their job, the number of uninsured persons grows by 85 (Rising Unemployment 2001). Medicaid could help to pick up some of these persons; however, in many states, Medicaid represents as much as 15 percent of the state budget (Medicaid Coverage 2001). In bad economic times, many states end up needing ways to cut state costs, especially since state sources of revenue such as income tax and sales tax are very sensitive to economic declines. If states respond to worsening fiscal situations by cutting Medicaid, the ability to secure public coverage to make up for lost insurance will diminish. These issues of the linkages between economic trends and access to health insurance and therefore to healthcare are very important. Although a country's overall economic health always plays a role in the amount of financing available for various services, because the United States depends on employment for coverage for many people and, unlike most European countries, generally does not have in place a system that guarantees access to health insurance or healthcare services, economic declines can lead to serious access problems for many people. At times, economic declines lead to more calls for reform of the U.S. healthcare system, but overall reform has been difficult to accomplish in the United States.

Healthcare Costs and Expenditures

One important factor to remember about how much healthcare costs in the United States and how we finance or pay for care is that the system for financing healthcare in the United States is not really a unified system. In Canada to the north, there are provincial budgets for healthcare, with a specified amount contributed by the Canadian federal government. In the United States, however, there is not a preset state or national budget for healthcare. We can present national data, but financing of healthcare services reflects the fragmentation in the U.S. system as a whole. How people pay for care varies by the insurance that people have and may also vary by type of provider and type of service.

One useful approach used by some analysts of our healthcare financing system is to talk of different categories of expenses: how much money is spent, where the money comes from (direct out-of-pocket, private insurance, government), and what it is spent on (fees paid to individual providers, to hospitals, for drugs or medically related supplies). National healthcare expenditures have grown at a rate substantially outpacing the gross national product (GNP) for most of the years since 1940, although there was a steadier rate of growth in the decade of the 1990s. Prior to World War II, only 4 percent of the nation's overall wealth each year was spent on healthcare. By 1960, this figure had increased only to 5.1 percent of the gross domestic product (GDP). Expressed in per-capita terms, the growth in health expenditures appears much larger, partially because this was a period of rapid economic growth. Per-capita expenses increased from $30 in 1940 to $143 in 1960 (Waldo, Levit, and Lazenby 1986; National Health Expenditures Tables 2001). These trends continued and accelerated in the next twenty years, as the percent of GDP spent on healthcare increased to 7 percent in 1970 and 8.8 percent in 1980. Per-capita expenses also continued to increase, going from $348 in 1970 to $1,067 in 1980 in constant dollars (Waldo, Levit, and Lazenby 1986; National Health Expenditures Tables 2001).

These decade-long figures actually mask important trends occurring within each decade. Health expenditures as a percentage of GNP and GDP were quite stable from 1950 to 1955, with more of an increase in the latter part of that decade (Kronenfeld and Whicker 1984). Major impacts on expenditures were created by the passage of Medicare and Medicaid in 1965 and the commencement of those programs' operation in 1966. After a brief period of wage and price controls from 1971 to 1973, the Medicare program expanded to more completely include the disabled, and costs rose again from 1973 to 1976. Then a voluntary effort to hold down healthcare costs ensued from 1976 through 1979 but gradually lost its effectiveness. During the decade of the 1980s, spending for healthcare continued to grow by almost all measures, with particular acceleration from 1986 to 1989 (Lazenby and Letsch 1990). By 1990, healthcare expenditures reached $695 billion, up to 12 percent of the GDP, an increase of about 10 percent from 1989 to 1990. This was an inflation rate substantially greater than the increase in overall GDP. In fact, the increase in the share of GDP spent for healthcare from 1989 to 1990 was the second-largest such jump since 1960 (Levit et al. 1991). One explanation for the large jump was the slowdown in the general economy. The percentage of GDP spent on health is very sensitive to overall economic growth because the denominator figure in percentage of GDP spent on health is a measure of overall output of the economy. The trends on per-capita expenditure are less dependent on overall economic trends. Per-capita expenditures also continued to increase during the decade of the 1980s, up to $2,737 by 1990 (Levit et al. 1991).

Costs continued to increase from 1990 to 1993. National health expenditures as a percentage of GDP remained relatively stable from 1993 through 1999, ranging from 13.4 percent in 1993 to 13.0 percent in 1998 and 1999 (National Health Expenditures Tables 2001; Cowan et al. 2001). One explanation for the small decrease in the percentage of GDP spent on healthcare in the late 1990s is the large increase in the GDP during that time period, a period of expansive economic growth. Other factors that helped to stabilize costs in that time period were one-time effects of managed care and some impact of federal legislation, such as the Balanced Budget Act of 1997, which limited growth in some of the government health spending programs. Per-capita health expenditures have continued to increase in the 1990s, going from the $2,737 figure in 1990 to $3,842 in 1996 and $4,358 in 1999 (National Health Expenditures Tables 2001; Cowan et al. 2001). The fact that per-capita expenditures are continuing to increase is one reason why experts are concerned that healthcare expenditures are increasing as a percentage of GDP in the first decade of the twenty-first century.

Figure 1.1 shows both where the nation's health dollars came from and went to in 1960 and in 1999. This allows a comparison of types of revenue sources and expenditures over time, before beginning a more detailed examination of, first, types of healthcare expenditures and then sources of revenue. A comparison of the sources of funds between 1960 and 1999 shows the

FIGURE 1.1
The Nation's Health Dollar—Where It Came From and Went in 1960 and in 1999

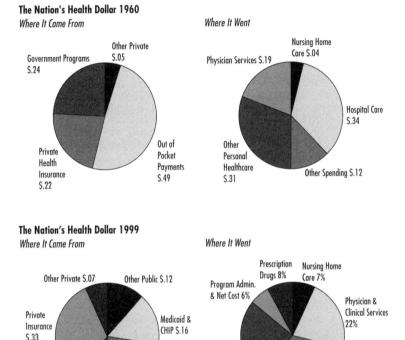

Source: Health Care Financing, Office of the Actuary. Health Care Financing Review. 22(4), Summer 2001.

greater influence of the role of government by 1999. Only 24 cents out of every health dollar in 1960 came from government programs. By 1999, government programs of all types contributed 45.3 cents out of every healthcare dollar. Almost 18 cents is being spent for Medicare, almost 16 cents for Medicaid and the CHIP program, and 12 cents for all other public programs. The importance of public programs has been increasing in almost every decade. For example, by 1990, government programs of all types covered 42 cents out of each healthcare dollar: 17 cents for Medicare, 11 for Medicaid, and the rest for other types of government programs both at the federal level and at state and local levels. Of course, in 1960, Medicare and Medicaid did not exist as federal programs, and the CHIP program did not exist in 1990. The next largest source of the healthcare dollars by 1999 was private health insurance, accounting for 33 cents of every healthcare dollar, the same amount as in 1990, but an increase from 22 cents in 1960. Far and away the largest source of the healthcare dollar in 1960 was out-of-pocket payments (that is, costs not reimbursed to the consumer). This category accounted for 49 cents, or almost half of all the healthcare dollar in 1960, but was only 15 cents by 1999, a continued decrease from 20 cents in 1990.

A comparison of where the healthcare dollar actually went in 1960 and 1999 reveals much greater similarities over the forty years. Hospital care was the largest single category of expense at both points in time, and consumed 34 cents of the healthcare dollar in 1960 and 33 cents in 1999, reflecting a small decline in the importance of expenditures in hospitals with the growth of outpatient care. This is a fairly new decline, since in 1990, 38 cents of the healthcare dollar was going to hospital services. The catch-all category of other spending in 1999 was the next largest single figure and covered such services as dental, other professional services, home health, durable medical products, and over-the-counter medicines. This category of spending accounted for 24 cents of each healthcare dollar. In earlier years, the categories were not identical, but the category of personal healthcare services was the second largest in 1960 (31 cents) and also in 1990 (23 cents), and included dental, home healthcare, drugs, and other nondurable products. Physician and clinical services took 19 cents of the health expenditure dollar in 1960 and 1990 and was up to 22 cents in 1999. Nursing-home care is one category that has almost doubled, taking only 4 cents of the healthcare dollar in 1960, 8 cents in 1990, and 7 cents in 1999, the small reduction being due to the growth in home health–based services (Levit et al. 1991; Office of National Cost Estimates 1990; Cowan et al. 2001). The importance of prescription drugs is indicated by its being given a separate category by 1999 and accounting for 8 cents of the national health dollar.

As the figures just discussed partially show, government expenditures as part of the healthcare system grew a great deal, especially from 1960 to 1990. During this time period, various reforms were implemented to try to control rising costs. The diagnosis-related group (DRG) prospective hospital-payment reform system was implemented by Medicare in 1983 as part of the Social Security amendments of that year and is explained in more detail in Chapter 2. The other major area of cost-related reform within the Medicare program in recent years was a new physician-payment approach begun in January 1992 and enacted as a way to deal with problems of rising costs in the Medicare program. One cost-related issue that has been receiving increased policy attention in terms of coverage for the elderly is drug costs. Since the failure of the Clinton healthcare reform efforts in the early 1990s, some policy experts have argued that drug costs for the elderly need to be covered in some way, perhaps through adding a prescription-drug benefit to Medicare, since prescription-drug costs now represent the fastest-growing segment of healthcare spending (Prescription Drug Trends 2001). Concern about rising drug costs may be the leading concern about the return of rising healthcare costs since 1999.

After six years of slower growth, estimates are that total national healthcare expenditures have increased yearly between 7 and 10 percent from 2000 to 2002 (Gardner 2001). Federal laws such as the Balanced Budget Act of 1997 included some caps on growth that restrained cost increases from 1997 to 1999. Increased numbers of patients in managed care plans in the 1990s also slowed cost increases. Few experts believe this will be the trend in the first decade of the twenty-first century. As the large baby-boom population begins to age, the pressures of care for that large group will help create increased costs, as will growth in new technology, new drugs, and changes in the organization of medical care.

Costs of health insurance have started to have double-digit increases since 1999 in some parts of the United States. During the economic expansion of the late 1990s, many employers absorbed health insurance cost increases. As the economic downturn began in late 2001, many employers planned to pass along such price increases, which ranged from 12 to 14 percent in large companies and 18 to 20 percent for small businesses (National Journal Examines Rises 2001).

Quality of Healthcare

Quality of care is inextricably intertwined with societal, professional, and patient expectations concerning the role of healthcare in society. Over the last twenty years, there have been several critical periods of more-detailed attention to what quality means and how to define it. In 1990, the Institute of Medicine defined quality as "the degree to which health services for individuals and populations increase the likelihood of desired health outcomes and are consistent with current professional knowledge" (Lohr and Schroeder 1990). Another way to think of this is that if providers deliver good-quality services, they are providing services in a technically competent manner, with good communication, shared decision making, and cultural sensitivity.

One older, classic assessment of quality, especially as related to patient care, is to divide aspects of quality into three components: structure, process, and outcome (Donabedian 1968; Brook, Williams, and Davis-Avery 1976; Donabedian, Wheeler, and Wyszewianski 1982). The simplest assessment in terms of availability of information is structure. Measures of structure of care relate to the personnel and facilities used to provide services and the manner in which they are organized. Licensure as a type of structural measure of quality is the most pervasive, most basic, and oldest quality-assurance approach. Licensure is used for most healthcare professions. Process measures typically reflect what was actually done to a patient, such as the numbers and types of procedures and laboratory tests that were performed (Donabedian 1968). One advantage of this approach over moving to outcome measures is that process of care, at least the technical aspect, is usually well documented in the medical record. One major caveat when using process measures is that the linkage between the process—what is done to a patient—and outcome is not always clear.

Outcome measures reflect the outcomes or impacts of care. Another way to think of outcome measures is as net changes that occur in a patient's health status as a result of the medical care received. Many experts now favor greater emphasis on outcomes to assess quality. This approach is not without controversy, however. One major concern is that many factors affect health, not just the care received, and too simplistic a focus on outcomes does not reflect these various factors. For example, if an elderly person is having problems hearing, it is not an appropriate quality outcome to say that the person has received good care only if her hearing is restored to the condition of her youth, since in most cases this is not possible with the current levels of health knowledge. Lost hearing often cannot be restored, but hearing aids can improve daily functioning. This would be the more appropriate measure of an outcome for visits of an elderly person to an ear specialist. Another concern is that for outcomes to be used as an indicator of quality of care, the outcomes need to be sensitive to different levels in the process or content of care, and not all outcomes are. For a patient with cardiovascular disease, an appropriate outcome might be enabling the patient to resume pain-free physical activities, if a person has coronary artery disease for which surgical procedures are appropriate. Some people, however, choose medication over surgery. Sometimes this is the correct choice for medical reasons due to other existing complications in the person's health. In other cases, it may be the choice of the patient to try medication first. In either case, the appropriate outcome measurement may need to be good control of pain rather than restoration of pain-free activities.

Major concerns about quality of healthcare are not new. In the first six months of 1988, four different public agencies released reports about issues in quality of healthcare (Becher and Chassin 2001). After this flurry of activity, physician organizations, quality experts, and legislators ended up agreeing that new efforts were needed. The initial most-visible result of this concern was the creation of a new federal agency to invest in research on the effectiveness of healthcare services and to develop practice guidelines to assist providers in improving quality. By 1994, this effort led to the creation of MEDTEP, the Medical Treatment and Effectiveness Program. One of the most important parts of this effort was the effectiveness research program known as Patient Outcomes Research Teams (PORTS). The effort has produced mixed results.

A number of recent articles have tried to summarize the new quality concerns in the United States, incorporating especially the critiques of the Institute of Medicine (2001) report that argued that physicians, nurses, and other health professionals are doing their best to provide good-quality care but that the current system does not reward innovation and communication. The 1999 report *To Err Is Human* found that more people die each year from medical mistakes than from highway accidents, breast cancer, and AIDS (Institute of Medicine 2001). This report created enormous concern among the public and controversy among U.S. physicians and physician organizations, many arguing that the public was becoming unnecessarily panicked about such problems. The more recent report has been received more favorably from within the medical profession and is raising among experts a number of questions about how to best think about quality issues.

One way to think about quality issues is that patients may suffer harm from three different types of quality problems (Becher and Chassin 2001). The first type of harm is if patients do not receive beneficial health services. The second is when patients undergo treatments or procedures from which they do not benefit. The third situation is when patients do receive appropriate medical services, but the services are provided inappropriately. A simple way to summarize these three types of problems is as underuse, overuse, and misuse. Health services research literature demonstrates that, on average, half of Americans do not receive recommended preventive care, 30 percent do not receive recommended care for acute conditions, and 40 percent do not receive care for chronic conditions. Similarly high rates of overuse have been demonstrated—about 30 percent for acute conditions and 40 percent for chronic conditions (Schuster, McGlynn, and Brook 1998). Studies of misuse are more complicated. Many have occurred in hospitals and one of the best known of these studies, the Harvard Medical Practice Study (1990), found that 1 percent of patients hospitalized in New York hospitals in 1984 had an injury from negligence. A different quality study using medical records from 1995 and 1996 at seven Veterans' Administration medical centers found that almost one-quarter of active-care patient deaths were possibly preventable by optimal care, and 6 percent were rated as probably or definitely preventable (Haywood and Hoffler 2001).

The 2001 Institute of Medicine report argues that the current U.S. healthcare system is a tangled, highly fragmented web that often wastes resources with unnecessary services and duplicated efforts. Possible solutions are to revamp the system to deal not only with the needs and values of patients but also to develop greater teamwork among health professionals and greater use of information technology. Some of the technological suggestions are better use of computers in the maintenance of medical records and information, automated medication-order entry systems to reduce human error, and the use of e-mail to facilitate communication between patients and doctors. A recent editorial in a major medical journal argues that more guidelines and better continuing education for physicians will be one key. Moreover, the development of better computer technology may make it possible for physicians to have handheld computers and computerized clinical-decision support systems in the future (Shaneyfelt 2001).

In the past decade, a number of specific studies have examined issues such as the type of organizations that deliver healthcare and the impacts that factor may have on quality. From a number of such studies have come recommendations that groups such as health maintenance organizations (HMOs) and preferred provider organizations (PPOs) continue to develop standardized performance measures. A number of these measures are currently in use, such as the Health Plan Employer Data and Information Set (HEDIS®) and the Consumer Assessments of Health Plans (CAHPS) (Kleinman 2001).

Some recent research on quality of care has explored the issue of settings of care. Research has demonstrated for some time that managed care settings can provide a quality of care as good as that provided in older fee-for-service settings; however, much of that research has been conducted on older, nonprofit managed care settings in which many of the physicians were in group and staff models. The more important question in today's managed care settings is whether quality of care varies between investor-owned and not-for-profit managed care settings. Compared to not-for-profit HMOs, investor-owned plans scored lower in a recent study on fourteen different quality-of-care indicators (Himmelstein et al. 1999). Investor-owned plans are more concerned about producing a profit for their investors and may skimp on some aspects of care to produce that profit. The domination of today's healthcare market by investor-owned plans may indicate growing concerns about quality. Some of these concerns about managed care have become part of the push among patients to have a patients' bill of rights, partially as a way to deal with quality-of-care issues and overall issues of patient satisfaction. Although different groups mean different things by the term *patients' bill of rights,* many versions would include allowing patients to sue an HMO in state court for denial of benefits or quality-of-care issues. A patients' bill of rights has been under serious discussion in the U.S. Congress since 1998 at least, but it has not yet been passed.

Quality concerns are not new to the health policy arena, nor are issues of access and cost. Issues of quality, cost, and access are intertwined, and will continue to receive attention as being among the most important issues facing the healthcare system of the United States. Although some legislation to deal with reform in these specific areas, such as a patients' bill of rights or legislation to cover drug costs for the elderly, may occur in the next few years, the examples just given are piecemeal, small reforms as compared to major overall healthcare system reform. The next chapter reviews the federal role in healthcare and periods of healthcare reform, with greater focus on major changes but some coverage of interim, smaller changes as well.

References

Aday, Luann, Ronald Anderson, and Gretchen Fleming. 1980. *HealthCare in the U.S.: Equitable for Whom?* London: Sage Publications.

Aston, G. 1998. Number of Uninsured Continues to Rise. *American Medical News* October 26: 5–6.

Becher, E. C., and M. R. Chassin. 2001. Improving the Quality of Healthcare: Who Will Lead? *Health Affairs* 20: 164–179.

Brook, R. H., K. N. Williams, and A. Davis-Avery. 1976. Quality Assurance Today and Tomorrow: Forecast for the Future. *Annals of Internal Medicine* 85: 809–817.

Budrys, G. 2001. *Our Unsystematic Healthcare System.* Lanham, MD: Rowman and Littlefield.

Cassil, A. 1997. Uninsured Patients Do Suffer, New Survey Reveals. *AHA News* 33 (48): 3.

Cowan, C. A., H. C. Lazenby, A. B. Martin, P. A. McDonnell, A. L. Sensenig, C. E. Smith, L. S. Whittle, M. A. Zezza, C. S. Donham, A. M. Long, and M. W. Stewart. 2001. National Healthcare Expenditures, 1999. *Health Care Financing Review* 22: 77–110.

Donabedian, A. 1968. Promoting Quality through Evaluating the Process of Patient Care. *Medical Care* 6: 181–202.

Donabedian, A., J. R. Wheeler, and L. Wyszewianski. 1982. Quality, Cost and Health: An Integrative Model. *Medical Care* 20: 975–992.

Eberhardt, M. S., D. D. Ingram, and D. M. Makuc. 2001. *Urban and Rural Health Charts, Health USA, 2001.* Hyattsville, MD: National Center for Health Statistics.

Freeman, H. E., R. J. Blendon, L. H. Aiken, S. Sudman, C. F. Mullinix, and C. R. Corey. 1987. Americans Report on Their Access to Health Care. *Health Affairs* 6 (Spring): 11–27.

Gardner, J. 2001. The 800 Pound Gorilla Returns. *Modern Healthcare* March 12: 5, 15.

Harvard Medical Practice Study. 1990. *Patients, Doctors and Lawyers: Medical Injury, Malpractice Litigation, and Patient Compensation in New York.* Cambridge, MA: Harvard University Press.

Haywood, R. A., and T. P. Hoffler. 2001. Estimating Hospital Deaths Due to Medical Errors. *Journal of the American Medical Association* 286: 415–420.

Himmelstein, D. U., S. Woolhandler, I. Hellender, and S. M. Wolfe. 1999. Quality of Care in Investor-Owned vs. Not-for-Profit HMOs. *Journal of the American Medical Association* 282: 159–163.

Institute of Medicine. 1999. *To Err Is Human.* Washington, DC: National Academy of Sciences.

———. 2001. *Crossing the Quality Chasm: A New Health System for the 21st Century.* Washington, DC: National Academy of Sciences.

Kleinman, L. C. 2001. Conceptual and Technical Issues Regarding the Use of HEDIS and HEDIS-Like Measures in Preferred Provider Organizations. *Medical Research and Review* 58: 37–57.

Kronenfeld, J. J. 1997. *The Changing Federal Role in U.S. Healthcare Policy.* Westport, CT: Praeger.

Kronenfeld, J. J., and M. L. Whicker. 1984. *U.S. National Health Policy: An Analysis of the Federal Role.* New York: Praeger.

Lazenby, H. C., and S. W. Letsch. 1990. National Health Expenditures, 1989. *Health Care Financing Review* 12: 1–26.

Lee, Phillip, and A. E. Benjamin. 1999. Health Policy and the Politics of Healthcare. In *Introduction to Health Services,* ed. Stephen J. Williams and Paul Torrens, pp. 439–465. Albany, NY: Delmar Publishers.

Levit, K. R., S. W. Lazenby, C. A. Cowan, and S. W. Letsch. 1991. National Health Care Expenditures, 1990. *Healthcare Financing Review* 13: 29–54.

Lohr, K., and S. A. Schroeder. 1990. A Strategy for Quality Assurance in Medicare. *New England Journal of Medicine* 322: 707–712.

Meckler, L. 2003. Thirty Percent in U.S. without Health Care Coverage in 2001–02. *Arizona Republic.* March 5, p. A17.

Medicaid Coverage During a Time of Rising Unemployment. 2001. Kaiser Commission on Medicaid and the Uninsured. http://www.kff.org/medicaid/4026index.crm (Accessed 1 January 2004).

Moyer, M. E. 1989. A Revised Look at the Number of Uninsured Americans. *Health Affairs* 8 (Summer): 102–110.

National Health Expenditures Tables. 2001. http://www.hcfa.gov/statistics/nhe/historical/ (Accessed 20 January 2004).

National Journal Examines Rises in Health Care Costs. 2001. *Kaiser Daily Health Policy Reports.* http://www.Kaisernetwork.org (Accessed 21 June 2001).

Office of National Cost Estimates. 1990. National Health Expenditures, 1988. *Health Care Financing Review* 11: 1–54.

Prescription Drug Trends: A Chartbook Update. 2001. http://www.kff. org/content/2001/3112 (Accessed 1 June 2001).

Rising Unemployment and the Uninsured. 2001. Kaiser Family Foundation. http://www.kff.org/uninsured/6011-index.cfm (Accessed 20 January 2004).

The Robert Wood Johnson Foundation. 1987. *Access to Health Care in the United States: Results of a 1986 Survey.* Special Report Number 2. Princeton, NJ: The Robert Wood Johnson Foundation.

Schuster, M. A., E. A. McGlynn, and R. H. Brook. 1998. How Good Is the Quality of Healthcare in the United States? *The Milbank Quarterly* 76: 517–563.

Shaneyfelt, T. M. 2001. Building Bridges to Quality. *Journal of the American Medical Association* 286: 2600–2601.

Steinmo, S., and J. Watts 1995. It's the Institutions Stupid: Why Comprehensive National Health Insurance Always Fails in America. *Journal of Health Politics, Policy and Law* 20: 329–372.

Thorpe, K. E., and C. S. Florence. 1999. Why Are Workers Uninsured? Employer-Sponsored Health Insurance in 1999. *Health Affairs* 12: 213–218.

Waldo, D. R., K. R. Levit, and H. C. Lazenby. 1986. National Health Expenditures, 1985. *Health Care Financing Review* 8: 1–21.

Wilensky, G. R. 1987. Viable Strategies for Dealing with the Uninsured. *Health Affairs* 6: 33–40.

Wilensky, G. R., and K. E. Ladenheim. 1987. The Uninsured. *Frontiers of Health Services Management* 4 (Winter): 3–31.

Wilson, R. W., and E. L. White. 1977. Changes in Morbidity, Disability, and Utilization Differences between the Poor and the Nonpoor. *Medical Care* 15: 636–650.

2

The Role of the Federal Government in Health and Earlier Healthcare Reform Efforts

This chapter will focus on the role of the federal government in health and how its role in the healthcare system has been expanding over the past 100 years in particular. As part of that review, we will focus on the efforts to pass more comprehensive healthcare reform in the United States and the movement along that path, much of which has occurred in the past 50 years.

Federal Involvement in Health (through the 1920s)

Most of the federal involvement in health in the United States occurred after 1900, and the bulk of the legislation actually was passed after 1950. Given the reserve clause (the provision in the Constitution reserving for the states all powers not explicitly given to the federal government) and the idea that health was mostly a state concern in the United States, early federal legislation focused on special groups for whom the federal government had special responsibilities. Most books mark the beginning of federal involvement in healthcare with the Act for the Relief of Sick and Disabled Seamen in 1798, also referred to as the Merchant Marine Services Act of 1798. This act provided health services for this special group of great interest to the young nation that depended on maritime trade. Shortly thereafter, legislation was passed to set up Merchant Marine Hospitals, the first major federally funded facilities to provide healthcare services. Other early federal government activities in health were legislation to impose quarantines on ships entering U.S. ports to prevent epidemics and legislation in 1800 to authorize federal officials to cooperate with state and local officials to enforce quarantine laws. In the period up to the Civil War in 1860, most federal health efforts focused on special groups, such as members of the military and the merchant marines, and drew the authority to deal with health issues from the constitutional power to raise and support armies and navies and the power to regulate foreign and interstate commerce. The types of issues that are most important in health policy and health reform today, such as special programs for the elderly and regulation of hospital and physician payment, were not considered issues for government involvement at that point in time. In addition, healthcare was much more of a small business at that time, with individual doctors setting up their own practices and negotiating with patients for fees. Some experts have called this era one when medicine was first a domestic enterprise and then became a commercial enterprise. During this period, government had little to do with the private transactions between medical practitioners and their patients except for redressing negligence (malpractice) and guaranteeing the sanctity of a contract, if a physician agreed to provide care for a group of patients (Starr 1982).

The Civil War was a major defining event in American history in many ways, and this included the role of the federal government in healthcare, although the changes in healthcare were slow and gradual in the period from 1865 to 1900. One of the critical aspects of the Civil War as an overall defining event for the United States was that gradually the federal government became more active in many ways. Some of the initial growth in the government's activity was in areas that were essential to the conduct of the war, such as raising an army. Other changes, however, became very important in healthcare. These included the beginning of federal aid to the states with the Morrill Act in 1862. Although this act focused on granting federal lands to each state and allowing the profits of those lands to be used for support of public institutions of higher education, these institutions became the land-grant colleges that hosted many programs in nursing, nutrition, and later, medicine. Just as important to healthcare policy as it has developed in the United States was the origin of the use of the general welfare clause of the U.S. Constitution to justify some federal actions. Today, that clause is the major justification for most federal involvement in healthcare, including most medical research, Medicare, Medicaid, and health training programs (Kronenfeld 1997).

In the Civil War and post–Civil War era, events that brought greater government involvement in health included immigration growth. As a result of the expanding immigrant population and a general fear of the spread of disease in the population, health legislation was passed that gave the surgeon general of the Marine Services Hospitals authority to impose quarantines to prevent the spread of diseases. The first general immigration law in 1882 included provisions to exclude immigrants for medical reasons and allowed federal inspectors and doctors on board ships to check for diseases. Some of the impact of the federal government in the healthcare area continued to be in collaboration with state programs, as states and cities began to establish departments of public health, often to deal with the growth of cities due both to foreign immigration and internal mobility. By 1902, a health act was passed that clarified some federal health functions by renaming the Marine Services Hospitals the Public Health and Marine Services and setting up a system of communications among state, territorial, and federal health officials. The surgeon general, the administrative head of the Public Health Service (PHS), was authorized to have an annual meeting of state and territorial health officers to discuss major health policies issues and concerns of the day. Early concerns were the control of trachoma (an eye disease), typhoid fever (a highly infectious disease transmitted by contaminated food and water), and nutritional-deficiency diseases such as pellagra (caused by a lack of niacin in the diet).

In the early 1900s, some of the major health policy issues involved reform not in the area of healthcare services delivery, since this was still viewed as an area of mostly private concern, but in the area of basic foods and drugs. Fueled by the investigation of journalists of that era into corruption in the production of drugs and foodstuffs, and by the success of novels that focused on this topic, such as *The Jungle* by Upton Sinclair that focused on the lack of sanitation in meat-processing factories, reformers pushed for a greater role for the federal government in food and drug safety. These concerns resulted in the passage in 1906 of the

Pure Food and Drug Act. Initially, this legislation focused on regulations about adulteration and misbranding of food and drugs and the control of substances within these products. This act has become the basis for most of the present-day regulation of testing, marketing, and promotion of both prescription and over-the-counter medication. Today, hot topics related to this area are whether tobacco can be considered a drug under this act and the control of herbal food supplements, and whether these need to be considered as "drugs" under federal law.

There were many groups in the United States pushing for various types of reform. The American Association for Labor tried to stimulate health insurance programs through state governments and through labor unions, and there were efforts to try out options such as sickness funds, which were being used in Germany in the early 1900s. Despite these reform attempts, other social changes prevented any of these options from becoming national legislation. World War I led to discrimination against German-based ideas, and sickness funds became viewed as too "German" a solution for the United States. Labor unions focused more on recruitment and their own growth and less on broader social programs and goals, especially in the period after World War I when the United States began a more conservative political era and labor unions felt threatened. In addition, pushing for a greater role for government in the provision of healthcare services became more difficult during the decade of the 1920s as suspicions of "socialist" types of programs grew and such programs were increasingly viewed as "un-American."

One of the major pieces of legislation passed in the latter part of this time frame was the Maternity and Infancy Act, also known as the Sheppard-Towner Act. Despite the conservative era, this legislation was passed in 1921 and provided grants to states to help them develop health services for mothers and their children. In addition to the specific content of this legislation, this idea of providing grants to states in the area of health has served as a prototype for later federal grant-in-aid programs. Although the goal of this program may seem simple and straightforward today, at the time, the program became very controversial. It generated criticism from conservative political groups and from the American Medical Association (AMA), which even described it as "an imported socialistic scheme." In addition to the controversy over its essential nature, the act also specified that the services had to be available to all residents of a state, regardless of race, and this provision was also controversial in the 1920s, given the reality of discrimination based on race in programs in many states. The act was not renewed in 1929, although some of the functions of this legislation were later restored as part of the Social Security Act of 1935 (Skocpol 1992; Wallace et al. 1982).

The Federal Role during the Depression, World War II, and the 1950s

Although major healthcare reform legislation was not passed during this era, there were movements to try to examine aspects of the healthcare system and major movements in the area of social services provision and reform. The Great Depression of the 1930s did lead to major federal actions in a number of areas, including banking, employment patterns in the federal government, business regulation, and the creation of the Social Security system. Major healthcare reform, however, did not end up being part of the legislation enacted as part of the Social Security Act of 1935. Some of the private reform groups that were considering broad social policy change as part of the reaction to the Depression did urge some national coverage of healthcare, as the Committee on the Costs of Medical Care did in its 1932 report. Nonetheless, President Franklin D. Roosevelt did not support adding a health insurance component to the Social Security Act, partially because of concern that this would arouse opposition from the AMA to the Social Security legislation. The Social Security legislation did create a social insurance program to provide economic security to the elderly and marked the initiation of the welfare state in the United States. In addition to creating Social Security for the retired worker, it created a means-tested social-assistance program, Old Age Assistance, for the aged poor, and categorically based welfare programs, such as the Aid to Dependent Children program (later changed to the Aid to Families with Dependent Children [AFDC]), which was the major general welfare program in the United States prior to welfare reform in the early 1990s. Over the years from 1935 to the 1970s, the welfare state expanded to include benefits for spouses and widows (1937), disability insurance for workers of all ages unable to work due to health concerns (1965), and Medicare and Medicaid, which will be discussed in more detail a bit later in this chapter (Quadagno 2002).

In addition to these individually based benefits, the Social Security Act of 1935 included a section (Title V) that provided grants to the states for maternal and child health services and child welfare services, and for services to crippled children. Another section (Title VI) authorized annual federal grants to the states for investigation of the problems of disease and sanitation, leading to the creation of new local health departments in many states and significantly increasing overall federal assistance for state and local public health programs. By the end of the 1936 fiscal year, about 175 new local health departments were created as part of this legislation (Kronenfeld 1997).

The program for crippled children represented a new thrust in federal legislation, since it included demonstration monies that became the precedent for amendments in later legislation that covered innovative program grants. The program included both comprehensive and preventive aspects, and covered all related medical care costs for crippled children or children with crippling conditions. Although this was a small, specialized group in the population, the program did represent the initiation of the federal government providing funds for direct care for a specialized group of the general population, not a group entitled to services due to their occupation and service to the country (such as being on active duty in the military, being a wounded veteran of a war, or in the merchant marine service).

The federal government led the way in other areas related to health and protection of the public health during this era. Consumer protection in the drug arena was expanded by the passage in 1938 of the Food, Drug and Cosmetic Act, requiring manufacturers to demonstrate the safety of drugs before marketing them. The role of the federal government in research was expanded through the Ransdell Act of 1930, which created the beginning of the National Institute of Health from the U.S. Health Service Hygienic Laboratory that had been established in 1901. The act provided money for buildings to house research activities, created a system of health fellowships, and authorized the acceptance of public donations for research on the cause, prevention, and cure of disease (Strickland 1978). This role expanded in 1937 with the creation of the National Cancer Institute that was authorized to award grants to nongovernment scientists and institutions, to provide fellowships for the training of scientists, and to fund direct federal government cancer research.

The federal government has a longer history of playing a major part in the direct provision of healthcare services for veterans. Although some limited efforts to provide services to seriously disabled veterans had begun at the end of World War I, the Veterans Act of 1924 codified and extended the role of the federal government in the provision of healthcare services to veterans. That act extended medical care to veterans not only for treatment of disabilities associated with military service but also for other conditions requiring hospitalization. Preference was given to veterans who could not afford private care. In 1930, the Veterans' Administration was created as an independent U.S. government agency to handle disabled soldiers and other veterans' matters, such as pensions.

The Roosevelt administration was interested in the consolidation of federal health functions as part of an overall administrative reorganization of the federal bureaucracy. In a 1939 reorganization, the PHS became a component of the Federal Security Agency (FSA). A major piece of legislation, the Public Health Service Act, was passed in 1944. This legislation created the Office of the Surgeon General, the National Institutes of Health (NIH), and the bureaus of medical services and state services. Activities that now came under the new federal agencies included research and investigation into selected diseases and health problems, working with state and local health agencies on projects including the collection of vital statistics (records on births, deaths, and other life events), and special grants for major diseases of the time, such as venereal disease and tuberculosis control. One of the major amendments to the Public Health Services Act was the Hill-Burton Amendment (also known as the U.S. National Health Policy Hospital Survey and Construction Act of 1946), which was the outcome of a major effort to reform healthcare services in the United States in the period after the end of World War II.

The Hill-Burton legislation was the first major amendment to the Public Health Service Act. This major piece of legislation was one of the first of several post–World War II federally funded health programs. Several different interpretations exist about the importance of this legislation and why it was passed. In the post–World War II era, many of the European countries passed legislation to reform their healthcare systems, as a reward to the general population for the toil of over five years of warfare on the

European continent, as a way to enhance concerns about social equity, and as a way to deal with the lack of attention given to civilian needs and civilian building during the wartime years. The United States had some similar concerns after the end of World War II. Very little hospital construction had occurred during the Great Depression and World War II, setting the stage for a need for federal legislation funding the building of hospitals. Many soldiers had received health services through the federal government during the war and hoped to continue to receive health services in the postwar era. Many laborers had received health insurance benefits in lieu of raises during the war, since providing health insurance was one way to reward workers during the price controls of the war. Within the United States, debate about a more comprehensive national health insurance system occurred, with Truman as president and the more liberal wing of the Democratic Party preferring that type of legislation. Organized labor, a major supporter of the Democratic Party at that time, was also in favor of more comprehensive healthcare reform. Some of the major support groups assumed significant reform was likely; however, important groups became vocal opponents of major reform, including the AMA and business interests. Republicans and the more moderate wing of the Democratic Party wished to have less-comprehensive legislation passed, although everyone recognized the need to increase the involvement of the federal government in healthcare and in meeting unmet healthcare needs. As a compromise once more-comprehensive legislation failed to pass, the Hill-Burton Amendments became the major postwar initiative of the federal government. Senator Lister Hill of Alabama was a crucial player in devising the strategy of having the government provide funds for hospital construction, with the assumption that the private marketplace would be able to meet the less-expensive needs of provision of health insurance.

The Hill-Burton Amendments provided grants to assist states to inventory their existing hospitals and health centers and to survey the need for the construction of additional health facilities. After state surveys were completed, grants for hospital construction were available. Funds for surveys and planning were allocated to the states based on total state population. Federal funding covered up to one-third of the total costs. Funds for construction were allocated through a formula based on population and per-capita income and again covered up to one-third of the costs.

Major healthcare changes and reform did not occur under the Eisenhower administration, or the years 1952 through 1960. In fact, Eisenhower campaigned against national health insurance in 1952. Given that, it is not surprising that the federal government's role in healthcare did not expand much during this time period, even though expansions of the federal role in other service areas did occur. It is interesting to realize that the same types of arguments about the importance of transportation and education to national defense used to expand the federal role in these areas under Eisenhower might have been applied to health, but they were not. For example, the federal highway program to build the interstate highway system was justified as a national-defense measure, as were federal funds to public-school systems to increase the competence of American students in science and math to keep up with the Russians after the success of the Russian space program in the launching of Sputnik in 1957. No such rationales were used to expand the federal role in healthcare services, perhaps because major supporters of the Republican Party, both the AMA and business groups, were opposed to major healthcare reform. The types of changes that did occur were modest, organizational changes. In 1953, reflecting the growth in the size and number of domestic social programs, the FSA was renamed and given department status as the Department of Health, Education and Welfare (DHEW). During the Carter administration in the late 1970s, a separate Department of Education was created, leaving federal health and welfare functions in the renamed Department of Health and Human Services (DHHS).

Kennedy-Johnson Years and Expansion of Federal Involvement in Health

Many major federal health policy developments occurred in this time period. The largest and most important was the passage of the Medicare and Medicaid programs as amendments to the Social Security Act. These programs will be discussed after briefly reviewing some of the other less major changes enacted. An important series of legislation related to health, but not to overall healthcare reform, was the 1962 amendments to the Food, Drug and Cosmetic Act. These amendments were partially passed as a reaction to the thalidomide disaster in Europe, in which a new drug turned out to cause serious birth defects in unborn babies, especially to their limbs. Although the drug was not approved for use in the U.S. market, the amendments were nevertheless a reaction to the situation and specified that a new drug needed to be effective, as well as safe, before it could be marketed in the United States.

A number of disease-oriented categorical programs that provided specific aid were passed, along with some programs aimed at specific regions of the country, such as the Appalachian Regional Commission, or at specific catchment (regional or disease) areas for health problems. Two important programs dealt with education for health professionals and mental health concerns. The Health Professions Educational Assistance Act of 1963 authorized direct federal aid mostly in the form of construction aid to medical, dental, pharmacy, and other health professional schools as well as scholarship and student-loan aid to the students in the schools. The grants were contingent on the schools increasing their first-year enrollment, and thus were part of a policy designed to address the concern about the lack of adequate numbers of health professionals. Increasing the supply of health-care professionals was one attempt, though not through direct provision of services, to deal with access issues. In the mental health area, the 1963 Mental Retardation Facilities and Community Mental Health Centers Construction Act provided assistance in combating mental retardation through grants for construction of research centers and grants for facilities for the mentally retarded. In addition, assistance was provided for construction of community health centers, and this proved to be a major effort at a time when many states were beginning the process of deinstitutionalization within state inpatient mental health facilities. The next year, in 1964, a separate Nurse Training Act was passed that authorized funding for construction grants to schools of nursing.

One interesting fact about many of the new programs enacted in this time period (of which this is only a partial list) is that few of them, even ones like Medicaid that we think of as part of a direct provision of services, were administered by the federal government. Medicare was one of the very few programs to deal with direct provision of services and to be administered at the federal level. Many of the other programs involved grants to states or to private health-related agencies. Grant-in-aid programs grew during the Johnson administration (excluding

Medicare and Social Security) from $7 billion at the beginning of the presidency of John F. Kennedy in 1961 to $24 billion in 1970 (Lee and Benjamin 1993). These programs became the prototypical type of involvement of the federal government in healthcare. Federal funds for biomedical research, health personnel development funds, hospital construction funds, healthcare financing, and a large range of categorical programs all grew in this time period, one of an expanding role for the federal government in healthcare.

In 1960, the introduction of a modest new program, the Kerr-Mills Act, expanded the federal government role in directly paying for health services. This legislation established a new program of medical assistance for the aged. Federal aid was given to the states to pay for medical care for medically indigent people sixty-five years of age and older. State participation was optional. The program became the forerunner of Medicaid and was implemented in twenty-five states before being superseded by Medicare and Medicaid.

The Social Security Amendments of 1965 established the Medicare program, the program of national health insurance for the elderly, through a new title, Title XVIII. They also established a special program of grants to the states for medical assistance to the poor through Title XIX (Medicaid). These programs went into effect in 1966. The debate over the enactment of these programs was fierce and focused on Medicare (with Medicaid being created almost as an afterthought and as an expansion of the Kerr-Mills program), and opposition was strong. The AMA led the opposition and not only lobbied Congress against the program but provided negative material about the program for doctors to place in their offices for patients to read. In some parts of the country, state and local chapters of the AMA suggested that doctors discuss their opposition to the program with patients to try to convince them to oppose the legislation and make their opposition known to Congress. The AMA opposed the program because of fears that it would lead to regulation of fees, a concentration of purchasing power, and a loss of physician control and autonomy. Although almost forty years and many other changes in healthcare have led to some of the results feared by the AMA, those results were not the initial impacts of the legislation. The program was passed largely as a result of the overwhelming electoral majority that the Democrats held after the sweeping victory of Lyndon Baines Johnson in the 1964 election.

In addition, LBJ's knowledge of Congress and his political skills in assembling a coalition of support were important, as was the presentation of data demonstrating that in the early 1960s, older Americans were disproportionately poor (45 percent of those sixty-five and over versus 13 percent of people between twenty-five and fifty-four) and could not afford to buy their own health insurance at that time.

The Medicare program is complicated to explain and has a number of major limitations in benefits, partially because at the time of passage, the goal was to create a program that provided health insurance coverage for the elderly that would resemble the typical insurance that many middle-class people had from their work-based health insurance plans. At that time, the use of copayments at the time services were received and deductibles (a set amount of expenses a person must reach before the plan would cover any costs) was common, so these were included in the plan. Coverage of medications was not common, and at this point is still not a part of Medicare, although there has been discussion over the past decade about passage of a drug benefit for Medicare. Many plans had slightly different provisions for hospital service and for medical care (doctor) services, and this type of differentiation in benefits was also created as part of the plan.

For the Medicare program, part A of the title provided basic protection against the cost of hospital and certain post-hospital services. Inpatient hospital service of up to 90 days during any episode of illness and psychiatric and inpatient services for up to 190 days in a lifetime were included. Extended care services, such as nursing-home care, were covered for up to 100 days during any episode of illness. Some home health services and hospital outpatient diagnostic services were covered initially (and these areas were expanded over time with new amendments).

Part B provided supplemental medical insurance benefits and was a voluntary insurance program, financed by premium payments from enrollees, along with matching payments from general Social Security revenues. Initially, enrollment was very high (over 90 percent), and even now, enrollment is generally above 98 percent, so that for realistic purposes, most elderly in the United States have both parts A and B of the Medicare program available to them. Physician and related services, such as X-rays, laboratory tests, supplies, and equipment, were covered, as were additional home health services. Both part A and part B physician and related services involved cost sharing by the Social Security recipient in the form of deductibles and copayments.

Claims and payment were not handled directly by the Social Security Administration but were paid through fiscal intermediaries such as large health insurance groups, especially Blue Cross-Blue Shield in many parts of the country. The Social Security recipient and the institutional providers, such as hospitals and nursing homes, were not directly reimbursed by the federal government but received payments from the fiscal intermediaries in their geographic area. Institutional providers had to meet conditions of participation, such as utilization reviews, that were aimed at ensuring a minimum quality of service. This program is an important departure from many earlier federal health programs in that it provides direct services to citizens, through a fiscal intermediary, but not through states and localities as has been the case with many other federal health-related programs. It is consistent with the model of Social Security, however, in which direct payments are sent to individuals from the federal government, except that because healthcare services are very expensive and bills come in slowly after services rather than quickly, the initial decision was to model payment after the major health insurance programs in the United States at that time, in which patients did not receive the money directly nor did they pay the healthcare provider, but rather healthcare providers sent bills to a third party (the insurance company or the fiscal intermediary), and then many of the bills were paid directly. Medicare, administratively, was more complex in some ways than the earlier portion of Social Security.

The Medicaid program is more complex in its administrative structure, although it follows a more standard pattern in healthcare of joint federal-state programs with a matching component in terms of funding. Medicaid was started as a program of medical assistance to public-welfare recipients, with participation on a voluntary basis by any particular state. Thus from the beginning there was variability in coverage and amounts of services funded across the states, as well as in participation. By 1970, all but one state, Arizona, participated in the program. But not all states included all possible components, such as a medically needed category. States had the option of extending eligibility to the medically indigent persons not on welfare who had a borderline-poverty level of income but earned too much to be eligible for federally subsidized welfare.

Under Medicaid, all states were initially required to provide at least five basic services: inpatient hospital care, outpatient hospital services, other laboratory and X-ray services, skilled nursing-home services, and physician services. A large number of optional services, such as optometric services, were available for states to consider as portions of the program. States could also opt to provide more-essential mental health coverage, ambulance transportation, and dental care, but they were not required to do so by the federal government.

Amendments to the Medicare and Medicaid legislation began only a few years after the initial passage, with many amendments having either the goal of extending the program or amount of services provided, or modifying the institutional eligibility requirements and reimbursement schedules. The 1967 amendments featured expanded coverage for durable medical equipment for use in the home, for podiatry services for nonroutine foot care, and for outpatient physical therapy under part B of Medicare, as well as adding a lifetime reserve of sixty days of coverage for inpatient hospital care over and above the ninety-day original coverage for any spell of illness. Certain payment rules were also modified in favor of providers. More significant changes were incorporated into the 1972 amendments. Some new services such as chiropractic services and speech pathology were added. Family-planning services were added to the list of basic Medicaid services. One set of changes increased eligibility in several important ways. Persons who were eligible for cash benefits under the disability provisions of the Social Security Act for at least twenty-four months were made eligible for medical benefits under the Medicare program. Additionally, Medicare services were extended to people who required hemodialysis or renal transplants for chronic renal disease by declaring them disabled and eligible for Medicare coverage under Title XVIII. This aspect became known as the ESRD (end-stage renal disease) program. Although this expansion represented a numerically small category of people eligible for Medicare coverage, the average medical expenses of these people and those in the disability category proved to be very high. At the time this provision was passed, some health policy experts believed this adding of various disease categories would be the model of expansion of Medicare as a form of universal health insurance coverage to more and more people. However, the expense of the program and changing times and attitudes have resulted in no further expansions of

Medicare based on specific disease categories. Moreover, the growing costs would increase concerns about federal costs and overall costs in the healthcare areas in years following this 1972 legislation.

Controversy, Contraction, and Unsettled Times in the Federal Role (1969–1979)

Attempting to divide the recent past into clear periods is always difficult. Although there are ways in which to divide the years from 1969 to the present (by presidencies or by shifts in political parties, for example), the rest of this chapter will discuss the Nixon administration and its failed attempt at major healthcare reform, along with some changes that occurred during the period; the contradictory trends of the Reagan presidency and the 1980s; and the failed attempt at major reform by the Clinton administration in the 1990s and the changes that occurred in the healthcare system in that decade, often less linked with federal legislation than in some of the earlier time periods. The period from 1969 through 1979 covers the policies and laws of the Nixon administration, the brief Ford administration, and the Carter administration—or two Republican presidencies (one in which the president was not elected to the office) and one Democratic presidency. One thing that has remained consistent since 1969 (given the failure of major healthcare reform in the first term of the Clinton presidency) is the controversy about the appropriate role of the federal government and the contraction in federal funding of healthcare in some ways (often due to the press of the growing federal debt and the need to constrain growth in all government programs, including healthcare).

During the Nixon and Ford administrations, considerable conflict developed between the branches of government, especially between the executive and legislative branches, over domestic social policy. President Nixon coined the term *New Federalism* to describe his efforts to move away from the categorical-programs focus of the Johnson years toward general revenue sharing. In revenue sharing, federal dollars are transferred into state and local governments (often through block grants) for many different purposes with fewer restrictions (strings) than was the case in specific-grant programs that often specified that funds should be spent on a certain type of program in the maternal and child health area, for example. Congress generally favored categorical grants with their detailed provisions and control, while Nixon pushed for revenue sharing and block grants to states. The Nixon administration also, in contrast to the Johnson administration, preferred actions in the private rather than the public sector. Categorical programs continued to grow, however, but in the health-care area, the huge growth of the Medicare and Medicaid programs swamped all other policy efforts. Some major policy initiatives outside of Medicare and Medicaid occurred in the 1970s. Health personnel policy over the decade of the 1970s shifted to more focus on areas with special needs rather than a focus on growth in all categories and places.

Most changes during the Nixon presidency and the brief presidency of Ford involved Medicare and Medicaid and attempts to control costs. These changes will be discussed in the following paragraphs. A number of the policies enacted in this period were designed to deal with rising costs through placing constraints on payments, reviewing care to be sure it was actually needed, and initiating changes in the organization of care delivery, with the first legislation encouraging the development of health maintenance organizations (HMOs), the forerunner of today's growth in managed care. Nixon had a goal of passing more-comprehensive national health insurance of some type in his second term, which began in 1972. In fact, at the time, many health policy experts believed major legislation might be passed, since the Democrats in Congress, led by Senator Edward Kennedy, were drafting such legislation and were in favor of it. A push from a Republican president made the passage of major reform appear possible, and both sides were interested in a compromise. However, during that term the Watergate scandal grew in importance and overtook all other legislative agendas. By the time Nixon resigned, the push for national health insurance had dissipated.

There were some important programs enacted in the health personnel and health facilities area, however. Federal subsidies of hospitals and other healthcare facility construction were ended, partially as a reaction to skyrocketing healthcare costs. In their place, some programs began to explore planning and regulatory mechanisms to control expansion of facilities. The National Health Planning and Resources Development Act of 1974, discussed in more detail under amendments to the Public Health Service Act, was one such program. Health personnel policies by the mid-1970s began to focus on specialty and geographic maldistribution of physicians rather than physician shortages, and by the end of this period there was a concern about physician oversupply.

As discussed in Chapter 1, costs of healthcare began to increase rapidly after the passage of Medicare and Medicaid, as access to healthcare services increased, and many services that some physicians and hospitals had provided as charity care became actual costs in the healthcare system, paid for by the federal government. Although it may appear contradictory, the 1972 amendments, along with the expansive provisions, also marked the first amendments to help control the growing costs of the Medicare program. Among the most important of the 1972 modifications was the establishment of Professional Standards Review Organizations (PSROs) to address problems of cost, quality case control, and medical necessity of services. Associations of physicians reviewed the professional activities of physicians and other practitioners within institutions. The use of PSROs by Medicaid was made optional in 1981, and later federal funding for PSROs was deleted, but the initial goal of the program was to ensure quality of care and also to control costs. Another modification linked to cost control was the addition of a provision to limit payments for capital expenditures by hospitals that had been disapproved by state or local planning agencies as a way to put some enforcement aspects into the health-planning mechanisms.

In 1976 through 1977, a major reorganization of the U.S. DHEW led to the establishment of a separate agency, the Health Care Financing Administration (HCFA), whose job was to assume the primary responsibility for implementation of the Medicare and Medicaid programs. This new agency took over functions that had been located in the Bureau of Health Insurance of the Social Security Administration (Medicare) and in the Medical Services Administration of the Social and Rehabilitative Services (Medicaid), and made issues of Medicare and Medicaid administration more easily centralized, but also more visible.

A major set of amendments dealing with antifraud and abuse in both Medicare and Medicaid was passed in 1977. These strengthened the criminal and other penalties for fraud, included federal monies for state Medicaid fraud units, and required uniform reporting systems for participating healthcare institutions. These were attempts to control costs and ensure quality.

A specific set of cost-control measures, the Medicare End-Stage Renal Disease Amendments, was passed in 1978 to deal with the ESRD program. Incentives were added to encourage the use of home dialysis and renal transplantation. A larger variety of reimbursement options for renal dialysis facilities was also included. Studies of the diseases and its treatment were also allocated, especially those focusing upon possible cost reductions in care for the disease.

There were few new policy initiatives in healthcare during the presidency of Jimmy Carter (1977–1980), both due to some lack of overall interest in the issue and due to lack of having policies enacted (such as failed attempts to have Congress enact new hospital cost-containment legislation). By the end of the Carter presidency, the climate for expansion in government programs was further diminished. By 1980, antiregulatory procompetition approaches were gaining in popularity at the national level, as were pushes to give more autonomy and control to state and local units, rather than the centralization of planning and regulatory programs that had been occurring in earlier decades. One major piece of legislation passed at the end of Carter's term was the 1980 Omnibus Budget Reconciliation Act, or OBRA 1980. This act included extensive modifications in Medicare and Medicaid, with 57 separate sections. Many sections focused on controlling costs, although some also expanded the services available, continuing the tradition of contradictions within the legislation, with some portions aimed at containing costs while other portions aimed at expanding services, which generally leads to at least modest cost increases. For example, the home health services provision of the Medicare legislation removed the 100-visit-per-year limit, but required that patients pay a deductible for home care visits under part B of the program. The goal of these changes was the encouragement of home care over the more-expensive institutional care. Some new services and providers were added, such as alcohol detoxification under part A of Medicare and nurse midwifery under Medicaid.

The series of amendments in Medicare and Medicaid set the stage for the Reagan administration efforts in health, many of which focused on the Medicare and Medicaid programs. The changes in the 1970s already demonstrated the differing concerns of cost containment, rationalization of care, expansion of some services, and the creation of new alternatives (such as the use of midwives for Medicaid that might have as its goal both an expansion and improvement of quality of care, along with cost containment). They also demonstrated how these two programs became more and more the focus of health-related legislation from 1980 forward. For example, coverage for some mental health services, services for the disabled, and alcohol detoxification all were added to the programs through amendments and became ways in which two programs initially aimed at physical healthcare for the aged and care for some groups of the poor became a way to address growing health and societal problems, such as alcohol abuse, drug abuse, and disability. Expansions, however, were never without costs, and cost increases, along with overall concerns about too large a role for the federal government in the lives of citizens and too high a growth of taxes, set the stage for a complicated period in health policy after Reagan was elected president in November 1980.

The Limited and Reactive Change of the Reagan-Bush Period (1980–1992)

Many of the important aspects of health changes and pushes for certain types of health reform in this period were linked to the overall policy directions of the Reagan administration and the Bush administration that followed it. At the time, the phrase "the Reagan Revolution" was often used to refer to an ascendancy of conservative values and goals, which included a questioning of the role of government and a belief that the private sector was better able to accomplish many societal goals. Although these notions were applied most strongly to economic policy, they also affected, at a philosophical level, ideas about how to deal with health problems, even though issues in healthcare ended up pushing certain reforms during this time frame. Among some of the themes in this time frame were a decline of planning, an interest in block-grant mechanisms, and a desire to control federal expenditures in healthcare.

Often, broader social and economic themes of an administration impact what happens in the healthcare sector, which then may drive the healthcare reform efforts of that administration. Under Reagan, there emerged a significant reduction in federal spending for domestic social programs, including the elimination of revenue-sharing funds that helped local areas fund various types of special programs, including health programs. Tax reduction for all became a major theme, and this led to significant increases in the national debt and consequently a decline in the capacity of the federal government to fund many domestic social programs, including health programs. Connected to the declines in availability of funds was a goal of decentralization of program authority and "devolution" of powers to the states. Block grants to states became one mechanism to accomplish this goal in many social programs, including healthcare. Block grants gave wide discretion to states in how funds were used and ended up increasing inequities across states. Although the Reagan administration did not accomplish its complete goal of consolidating all of the twenty-six public health programs into two large block grants, it did succeed in having twenty programs combined into four block grants, while six remained categorical.

Deregulation was one overall Reagan administration goal. As applied to health, this eventually resulted in the end of federal health-planning efforts, since the Comprehensive Health Planning and Public Health Service Amendments of 1966 were not renewed in the 1980s. Given the Reagan political philosophy that government regulations should be reduced, funds for health planning were gradually eliminated. In fiscal year 1981, before Reagan was president, the entire health-planning program was funded for $126.5 million. By fiscal year 1983, the funding level was reduced by 54 percent, and the presidential budget had requested the removal of all planning funds. The Tax Equity and Fiscal Responsibility Act (TEFRA) of 1982 led to the dropping of requirements for local planning agencies known as Health Systems Agencies (HSAs) and made the use of the quality-control agencies known as professional review organizations (PROs) optional in hospitals for patients funded by Medicare and Medicaid, whereas it had previously been required (Kronenfeld 1997). From a philosophical perspective, the deregulatory attitude of the Reagan administration was grounded in a belief that the regulatory costs exceeded the regulatory benefits (Williams and Torrens 1993).

Consistent with its philosophy, a reform enacted during the Reagan administration was to reduce the role of the federal government in health personnel planning and training. Funds were cut drastically for new scholarships that had been provided through the National Health Service Corps to encourage physicians and nurses to work in rural, underserved areas after their professional training was completed. Grants to health professional schools based on their enrollment (known as capitation grants) were either totally eliminated or cut back drastically. Student-loan programs in the health professions were cut in half from fiscal year 1982 to fiscal year 1985.

Some of the reforms in healthcare appear partially contradictory. Funds were eliminated for HMOs, despite the emphasis in the Reagan administration on a procompetition model of healthcare. Under this model, HMOs were one mechanism for care delivery and a part of increasing competition in healthcare, since multiple HMOs in the same geographic area would be able to compete for customers. The stance of the administration, however, was that federal funds were unnecessary to stimulate this competition and that private market forces would be sufficient to facilitate HMO growth.

Some legislative actions did not have major budgetary implications but rather were focused on issues relating to quality of care. One of the last major pieces of general health-related legislation before the election of President Clinton was the OBRA 1990 (Omnibus Budget Reconciliation Act) legislation, passed under Bush. This legislation included the Patient Self-Determination Act as part of that OBRA 1990 legislation. Healthcare institutions participating in Medicare or Medicaid (virtually all medical care institutions) had to provide all patients with written information on policies regarding self-determination and living wills. Additionally, facilities had to determine whether patients had advance medical directives. The goal for the legislation was to increase discussion and consideration of the conditions under which a person might no longer wish to receive many medical services. Although institutions are complying with the legislation by having patients sign additional pieces of paperwork, it is less clear that the requirement increases the real level of discussion about these issues.

The majority of the reforms to the healthcare system during this period related to the Medicare and Medicaid programs, partially because these programs had become such an important part of overall expenditures for healthcare. The Reagan administration supported major legislative changes in Medicare and Medicaid. The majority of both proposed and enacted changes in Medicare were attempts to deal with the problem of healthcare costs. The Omnibus Budget Reconciliation Act of 1981 (OBRA 1981) was massive in its impact and number of changes to

Medicare and Medicaid, with forty-six different sections relating to the programs. A number of things were deleted from coverage. This reduction in covered services included eliminating the coverage for alcoholic detoxification facilities and the removal of occupational therapy as a basis for entitlement for home health services. The part B deductible on Medicare was also increased. In 1981, matching federal Medicaid payments to the states were reduced by 3 percent in fiscal year 1982, 4 percent in fiscal year 1983, and 4.5 percent in fiscal year 1984, although the cutback could be lowered by 1 percent in each fiscal year if a state operated a qualified hospital cost-review program, had an unemployment rate over 15 percent of the national average, and had an effective fraud and abuse recovery program. Prior to 1981, Medicaid required states to offer recipients freedom of choice in the selection of providers. After 1981, states could apply for waivers of the freedom-of-choice requirements and could require Medicaid recipients to receive care from a specially designated pool of providers, the beginning of mandatory Medicaid HMOs for some recipients.

The TEFRA 1982 made a number of important changes in the Medicare and Medicaid programs. Copayments for basic services, previously prohibited by federal statute, were made optional for states under the 1982 amendments for Medicaid. The regulations on acceptable error rates for Medicaid were tightened. For Medicare, hospice services were added as a covered service. The most important changes were part of an effort to control rising costs. The TEFRA set a limit on how much Medicare would reimburse hospitals on a per-case basis and limited the annual rate of increase for Medicare's reasonable charges per discharge.

Even-larger changes in the reimbursement policies of Medicare were passed in 1983. The Medicare Prospective Payment System (PPS) was created, which based payments to hospitals on predetermined rates per discharge for diagnosis-related groups (DRGs) as contrasted to the earlier cost-based system of reimbursement that had been in place since the initial passage of the Medicare program. In this act, Congress also directed the administration to study physician-payment reform options.

The DRG payment system was a major break with how payment had occurred in the past and was also a complex system that was regulatory in content. The federal government listed detailed regulations that explained how the new system would work and forced hospitals that received Medicare funds (basically all hospitals in the United States) to completely rethink and redesign payment systems. For an administration committed to competition and the private marketplace as the determinant of the distribution of healthcare resources, this regulatory approach seems quite surprising. The Reagan administration, in this case, demonstrated that healthcare issues were less critical to it than many other policy areas. If rising costs in healthcare were going to make tax cuts and other policy goals of the Reagan administration impossible, then a regulatory strategy to hold down healthcare costs was acceptable.

The DRG prospective hospital-payment reform system did help to contain the growth in hospital costs to some extent. Most hospitals in the United States are reimbursed by Medicare as part of this system, although psychiatric, rehabilitation, children's, and long-term care hospitals have a somewhat different arrangement. The rate of growth in annual hospital expenses did slow for a few years after the implementation of the DRG system, but then the rate of growth began to increase again. Some of the early fears about the implementation of this system were that hospitals would discharge sick patients too quickly and lead to unnecessary readmissions. There was some evidence that this occurred during the early phases of the DRG payment system (Gay et al. 1989). Some reforms in payment for readmissions have occurred, so that readmissions within too short a period of time no longer generate the start of a new DRG payment for that hospitalization. Overall, the system has led to shorter lengths of stays. Lengths of stays have dropped, about 0.9 days in 1984 and 0.6 days in 1985 compared to an average drop of 0.2 days per year from 1967 to 1983 (Koch 1988). For the majority of patients, it no longer appears that access to needed care has lessened under DRG reimbursement (DesHarnais et al. 1987), and hospitals have shifted more care into outpatient settings. By the early 1990s, it was clear that the DRG system led first to a decline and then a stabilization in inpatient hospital use from 1987 on, while outpatient hospital care continued to increase, as did costs for physician care (Edwards and Fisher 1989). Thus the actual impact of the payment reform system on total costs was less than hoped. Many would agree that the DRG payment system has been a success in the United States, and this approach to payment has been adopted or discussed for adoption by a number of other countries, such as Australia, Belgium, Norway, Sweden, and Portugal (Wiley 1992).

As with so many reforms that affect only one payer and one type of service, there is much room for hospitals and other providers to learn how to "game" the system, that is, maximize revenue given the new rules. Many analysts contend that piecemeal reforms of the healthcare system generally lead to disappointing results after a few years.

In 1984, the Deficit Reduction Act (DEFRA) continued to make changes in both payment of hospitals and payment of physicians. Further amendments for the rest of the decade also made changes in both areas, as well as other overall policy shifts. First, this section will discuss hospital payment and general policy changes, and then issues in reform of physician costs. The DEFRA legislation placed a specific limit on the rate of increase in the DRG payment rates in the following two years. The Graham-Rudman-Hollins Act of 1985 established mandatory deficit-reduction targets for the five subsequent years. This had a significant impact on the Medicare program, leading to cuts in payments to both hospitals and physicians. The Consolidated Omnibus Budget Reconciliation Act (COBRA) of 1985 adjusted payments under Medicare for hospitals that served a disproportionate share of poor patients. Hospice care was made a permanent part of the program. PPS payment rates were frozen at 1985 levels for part of the year as a way to hold down healthcare costs, and payment to hospitals for indirect costs of medical education was modified. Further, more-technical modifications continued in 1986 through 1989.

Although many of the earlier changes were attempts to control costs, some reform was directed at improving quality and access to care, even in the cost-conscious Reagan era. In the Medicaid program, expansion of services was included, with states being required to cover eligible children up to age six, with an option up to age eight. Additionally, the distinction between skilled nursing facilities and intermediate-care facilities was eliminated, and a number of features designed to enhance the quality of care in nursing homes were included.

A major potential reform, the Medicare Catastrophic Coverage Act, was passed in 1988 that included a large expansion in Medicare benefits. This act included provisions to add coverage for outpatient prescription drugs, respite care, and a cap on out-of-pocket spending for copayments by the elderly. The new benefits were to phase in over four years and be paid for by premiums, including an income-related supplemental premium, charged to

Medicare enrollees. This legislation was a major departure from previous policy making in the area of social insurance, because the expanded benefits were to be funded entirely by those who were current beneficiaries, and there would be overt redistribution among them. Despite being supported at the time by President Reagan, majorities in both houses of Congress, and the nation's largest senior-citizen interest group, the American Association of Retired Persons (AARP), the legislation was repealed less than eighteen months later after enormous criticism (Himmelfarb 1995). Wealthier elderly persons objected to paying the income-tax surcharge and additional premiums. Many average-income elderly persons were upset to discover that what they considered the biggest need in the catastrophic coverage area, coverage for nursing homes and long-term care costs, was not included. Others failed to grasp what the extensions of the program would provide to them, even though the legislation would have benefited all of the elderly without supplemental coverage and might have provided those benefits at a lower cost to many of those paying for that coverage. As is often the case in politics and public opinion, perceptions matter, at times, more than facts. The pressure on Congress from both elderly constituents and interest groups increased, and the legislation was repealed before most provisions were implemented.

The other major area of reform within the Medicare program was to control physician costs, ultimately through a new physician-payment approach. In 1984, the DEFRA temporarily froze increases in physician payment under Medicare and mandated that the Office of Technology Assessment study alternative means of paying for physician services as a way to guide reform of Medicare. The act also created a differential between two classes of physicians, participating and nonparticipating, under Medicare. The OBRA 1987 reduced physician fees for twelve "overvalued" procedures and built in higher fee increases for primary care than for specialty care.

The major reform in physician payment was in the OBRA 1989 legislation. The HCFA was directed to begin implementing a resource-based relative value scale (RBRVS) for reimbursing physicians under the Medicare program with a four-year phase-in period. The new system began in January 1992.

Previously, physicians had been paid on the basis of what their charges were for various services. In the studies prior to the development of the scales, how long it took physicians to perform various kinds of tasks was determined. Each service was assigned a relative weight based upon three geographically adjusted values for work, practice costs, and malpractice premiums. Thus new payment schemes were created related to the time and resources used. For the final application, a scale of relative weightings or relative values was formed as the basis of the new physician-reimbursement system for Medicare patients (Hsiao et al. 1988; Hsiao et al. 1990). Physician groups launched protests in June 1992 when the initial draft regulations were first released. The AMA was so upset that they threatened to seek congressional action to change the proposed new system of reimbursement (McIlrath 1991a). Physicians argued that the reimbursement scheme was not fair and that transition rules were particularly inappropriate (McIlrath 1991b). Based on the complaints in reaction to the initial drafts, the HCFA did revise the rules somewhat. Whereas the initial regulations would have increased slightly the fees paid to generalist physicians and decreased the fees paid to specialists, negotiations with various groups from organized medicine including the AMA were used as a basis for some modifications.

One other reform included in the OBRA 1990 legislation was aimed at simplification of Medigap policies, those policies that the elderly buy to supplement their Medicare coverage. Most of these policies cover some of the drug costs and the copayments that are required by the current structure of Medicare. Before this legislation, Medicare beneficiaries had a choice of hundreds of Medigap policies, with widely varying benefits that were difficult to compare from one plan to the next. Because of the new legislation, by July 1992 all Medigap policies had to conform to one of ten standardized packages developed by the National Association of Insurance Commissioners (NAIC). In a study of the impact of this legislation, most consumers have picked plans that offer the most coverage of Medicare's patient cost-sharing requirements. Fewer consumers have picked the more expensive plans that offer additional benefits such as preventive care, at-home recovery, and prescription drug coverage.

The Medicare and Medicaid reforms, especially the major ones on payment of hospitals and physicians, as well as other changes in the Reagan-Bush years, yielded mixed results as viewed from a policy perspective. Although the elimination of regulatory approaches was one goal of these administrations, this was accomplished only in the health-planning area. Especially in

Medicare and Medicaid, the Reagan and Bush administrations used regulations to limit hospital reimbursement and physician fees in the Medicare program. Even on a smaller scale, they used regulation to control the variety of Medigap policies offered so as to protect elderly consumers from purchasing worthless policies. Despite the talk about stimulation of procompetition approaches, HMOs did not receive financial incentives and encouragement, and growth in this area was modest in many sections of the country during this twelve-year period. The largest impact on health services during this time period came from the dramatic reduction in federal fiscal capacity due to tax cuts, the growing federal deficit, and initial attempts to control the deficit. Congressional efforts focused on controlling cost increases through regulation rather than procompetitive approaches. Even though the numbers of uninsured had been increasing in this twelve-year period, access concerns were not a major policy focus; rather, most attention was given to controlling healthcare costs, partially because healthcare spending outpaced the growth of most of the economy through this time period. As has often happened with a shift in political administration, the view of major problems in the health policy area also shifts gradually. The beginning of the Clinton administration arrived at a point of growing concerns about access to care, as well as costs and attempts at large reforms, as discussed in the next section.

The Clinton Administration, Failure in Major Healthcare Reform, and the Current Situation

There were a number of major pushes toward reform that were part of the policy climate in early 1993 at the time of the first inauguration of President Clinton, the time when his push for major healthcare reform began to seriously take shape. The factors behind the pushes toward reform included (1) changes in health insurance coverage within the United States; (2) fear of unemployment and the overall economic climate and its linkages to healthcare; (3) the political pushes from within the Democratic Party and those advising the presidential candidate that healthcare might be an important issue for winning an election;

and (4) the policy goals of the president that focused on his desire to pick a major issue in American society and have a lasting impact upon that issue, both to help achieve the political goals of a second term and to help achieve broader goals of having a presidency that makes an important impact upon American society.

Having good health insurance coverage is one of the most basic indicators of access to healthcare services in the United States. After the introduction of private insurance in the United States, issues of lack of health insurance coverage became a problem of special groups, such as the aged, the poor, and more recently the unemployed. Medicare helped to deal with access problems for the aged, and Medicaid helped for some of the poorest. Although there is a range of estimates about the numbers of people uninsured and underinsured in the United States from the early 1980s on, most sources agree that there has been an increase in the numbers of uninsured since the late 1970s (Access to Health Care 1987; Andersen and Davidson 1996). In the late 1970s, the best estimates were that 25 to 26 million people in the United States were without healthcare insurance. This was about 13 percent of the population under 65. The numbers of uninsured grew in the 1980s. Recent estimates range from a low of 22 million to a high of 37 million by the late 1980s. In a review of statistics from 1980 to 1993, one source estimates that the uninsured population increased from 13 to 17 percent from 1980 to 1993 (Andersen and Davidson 1996). Medicaid coverage was made available to more of the population (from 6 percent to 10 percent) but coverage by private health insurance became available to less of the population (from 79 to 71 percent). The proportion covered by private health insurance decreased for every age group, and the decline was especially noticeable for children under 15.

Critical to understanding how some groups of people have no health insurance in American society is the realization that most private health insurance in the United States is purchased through employer-based group insurance policies. This type of insurance represents about 85 percent of all private coverage. One major factor in the increase in the number of uninsured persons during the 1980s and early 1990s was the growth in unemployment in the early 1980s and again in the early 1990s. There is another group of people with no insurance—those with a history of serious medical problems. Many people with serious health problems do maintain health insurance coverage as long as they keep their jobs. If they lose their current jobs due to the general economy or their health but can still work, they may experience problems in finding employment due to their health. Although people who are medically uninsurable are a small part of those without health insurance, they are important because they are very high utilizers of health services. Studies have estimated that .5 to 1.0 percent of the U.S. population is currently "medically uninsurable."

It is never clear at the time what events will push a new or revised political agenda forward. In 1990, while most of the trends described in the previous two sections about rising numbers of Americans without health insurance and growing fears of the middle class about not having health insurance due to changes in the economy were already known, nevertheless neither health policy experts nor politicians considered it politically feasible to talk about major governmental reform in healthcare (Skocpol 1995). Certainly some major pressures were building. The *Journal of the American Medical Association* published a special issue in 1991 that focused on the issue of caring for the uninsured and underinsured. But while these kinds of actions resonated with the health policy community, they did not lead to broad discussion among the public. Then, unexpectedly, in the summer of 1991, the type of event described by policy experts as a "focusing event" occurred (Kingdon 1984). Following the tragic death of Senator John Heinz in an aviation accident, the relatively unknown (but long-time political activist) Harris Wofford became the Democratic senatorial candidate in a special election in Pennsylvania. He aired a television commercial during the campaign that argued: "If every criminal in America has the right to a lawyer, then I think every working person should have the right to see a doctor when they're ill." This spot resonated with the public, and led to a focus in his campaign on calls for national health insurance. Wofford managed to defeat his opponent, and the Democratic Party began to realize that access to healthcare was an issue on the minds of the public.

During the Democratic primary debates, health insurance was a topic of major discussion. Several of the candidates developed well-thought-out, detailed proposals about health reform. Although Clinton was not particularly identified with health issues in the early days of the primary campaign, after being pushed by rivals, he released a ten-page-long healthcare policy paper during the New Hampshire primary debates in January 1992. In the summer of 1992, when it was clear that Clinton had won the Democratic nomination for the presidency, Clinton and his aides realized that healthcare could be an important issue in the upcoming election. In his acceptance speech at the Democratic convention in Madison Square Garden in 1992, Clinton vowed "to take on the healthcare profiteers and make healthcare affordable for every family." This rhetoric provided a sense of direction and commitment to the public at large, but the campaign advisors were leery of providing more details. Campaign polls showed that voters wanted the system changed, but were not certain what changes would help them (Johnson and Broder 1996).

After Clinton won election in November 1992 the immediate issue was how important healthcare reform would be in his administration. For a politician who thought of himself as a policy wonk or detailed policy expert, who was concerned about how presidents are viewed by history, and who wanted to leave a lasting impact on the country, healthcare reform was the most challenging issue on the domestic agenda and the one that would impact the greatest number of people. It was an issue in which everyone in the country shared some concern, as contrasted with welfare reform, which would impact a more limited number of people in the country. Five days after the inauguration, President Clinton announced the formation of the president's Task Force on National Health Reform. The job of the task force was to prepare healthcare reform legislation to be submitted to Congress within 100 days of beginning in office. Hillary Rodham Clinton, wife of the president, was named head of the task force. Despite advice against the creation of the commission, against tackling overall healthcare reform as one big piece, and against appointing his wife as the head of the commission, Clinton moved ahead with his plans.

Many of his former aides argue that, in some ways, Clinton's own intellectual capacities worked against successful healthcare reform. He was not intellectually inclined to follow the advice of more piecemeal reform efforts. He wanted a large impact, and he saw the interconnections between health problems. He wanted to tackle the entire issue. A number of books and articles have now reviewed, in greater detail than is possible here, how this effort at major healthcare reform faltered (Starr 1994; Blendon et al. 1995; Johnson and Broder 1996; Yankelovich 1995). These analyses point to difficulties with the commission, problems with understanding the political process, weaknesses in overall Democratic strength and support of the plan, and problems in presentation of the issue to the public and communication to the general public, as well as the lack of coalescing important interest groups to lobby for the plan, especially since groups opposed to the plan did develop effective lobbying and public-communication approaches.

Some experts argue that one of the important flaws in the process was the lack of a real public debate over and public consensus regarding the issues (Yankelovich 1995; Blendon et al. 1995). Daniel Yankelovich, a public-opinion expert, has argued that both the defeat of the catastrophic-coverage plan for the elderly in 1989 and the defeat of the Clinton healthcare reform plan in 1994 reflect a "massive failure of public deliberation" (Yankelovich 1995, 8). He argues that the nation's leadership class (including leaders of medicine, industry, education, the legal profession, science, religion, and journalism) does not talk effectively with the public. All the groups crafting the healthcare reform plan were from this leadership class, and the average American did not understand it and what it meant for them. Because of this, Yankelovich argues that the plan lost public support because its opponents found it easy to raise public fears about a plan people did not understand. In support of this argument, Yankelovich demonstrates that public knowledge about the plan decreased over time. Right after Clinton presented his health address to the nation, only 21 percent of the public said they knew much about it. But, instead of these numbers increasing over time, by the next month, the numbers had decreased to 17 percent, and they continued to fall up to the time that Congress considered the legislation in August 1994, when only 13 percent of Americans felt they were very well informed about the debate in general (Yankelovich 1995). If the support of the public helps to push major reforms, the public must understand some aspects of the plan, at least enough to form an opinion about the proposed plan.

If Yankelovich is correct that the defeat represented massive failure of public deliberation and was linked to a lack of public understanding about the plan (or plans as they changed), what does public-opinion data show about overall support for the plan? Blendon and colleagues (1995) also have reviewed public-opinion data and concluded that within a twelve-month period, support for the Clinton plan fell from 71 percent to 43 percent. Although some of this loss of support was attributed to substantive choices and specifics of the plan, some is attributed to a lack of communication with the public, especially the middle class, who became convinced the plan benefited the poor more than themselves (and perhaps was part of the reason that some Democratic politicians became convinced that they were going to lose control of the Senate over the issue of healthcare reform). To make the process more difficult, the general public also distrusted the ability of government to do what is right most of the time, an important change from the public's attitudes in the 1960s when Medicare and Medicaid were enacted. Thus, building public support is harder in the 1990s, but no less important, especially for a president in a relatively weak position as regards congressional majorities.

Other types of criticism and explanations for failure based partially on process and partially on content focus on the whole development process and the presentation of the reform plan by the president. One historian who has reviewed the failure of the Clinton healthcare reform plan from the vantage point of historical experience has argued that the entire process used by the Clinton administration allowed comprehensive healthcare reform to be too defined as a purely presidential initiative, and did not allow for either public involvement and discussion of trade-offs or for negotiations with Republicans who supported the general goal but did not want to contribute to the triumph of a new Democratic president (Heclo 1995). In comparison to the success that President Johnson was able to accomplish in passing his War on Poverty legislation including Medicare and Medicaid, President Clinton's reform also came to be viewed as a test of the president's personal popularity, but Clinton lacked the large congressional majorities that allowed Johnson to successfully have legislation passed. (In addition, Clinton enjoyed neither the understanding of congressional operations that Johnson had gained from his decades of service in the Senate nor Johnson's strong personal contacts with senators).

Not all of the problems of process were due only to missteps by the Clintons. According to more recent reports, some conservative experts had concluded that successful passage of a Clinton healthcare plan would provide enormous trouble for the success of Republicans in the next sets of congressional and presidential elections. Bill Kristol, who worked for the conservative think tank The Project for the Republican Future, argued that congressional Republicans should work to kill, rather than amend, the Clinton plan. He argued that doing so would enhance Republican chances of winning Congress and of becoming the majority party, dovetailing with the views of Newt Gingrich whose "Contract with America" would become a theme for the 1994 elections (Johnson and Broder 1996). This strategy became a reality in the plans of the Senate Republicans, who blocked the discussion of healthcare bills, as well as in the statements of Gingrich on the House side and his ability to first delay the health bill and then link its consideration to defeats in other areas.

The 1994 congressional elections had the potential to be major transforming elections in the United States. Republicans gained a majority in both houses of Congress, taking control of the House of Representatives for the first time in forty years. Gains were large, with fifty-two seats gained in the House and eight in the Senate. Although the healthcare issue was not the only reason the Democrats did poorly in the election, the defeat of healthcare reform certainly played a role in the defeats. One study (Blendon et al. 1995) that examined public-opinion survey data at the time of the election and national Election Day exit surveys determined that most voters did not choose a candidate for Congress based on healthcare or even other national issues. Only 22 percent of voters said that stands on national issues were one of the most important factors, as contrasted with the candidate's experience, character and ethics, and political party. However, if voters were asked about concerns with specific issues, healthcare became more important. Looking at data from Election Day surveys, healthcare was rated as number one in two of the surveys and tied for fourth in the third. Another question asked voters to name their top priorities for the new Congress. Only two surveys asked this question, and in both, healthcare was listed as number one. In examining issues of importance to voters and programs people support, voters were more in favor of providing health insurance to certain "deserving" groups. Voters favored covering children first and then people who were uninsured. About half were willing to pay a modest increase in taxes or health insurance premiums to see some changes made in the healthcare system. Traditional Social Security and healthcare programs received wide support. Only 17 percent were willing to see cuts in Social Security or Medicaid as ways to deal with deficits, and even fewer (7 to 8 percent) were willing to see cuts in Medicare and veterans' benefits, versus much higher support for welfare cuts in programs such as food stamps, public housing, and AFDC.

Given the Republican control of both houses of Congress, legislators did propose a balanced budget by 2002 with large cuts

(20 percent in Medicare and 30 percent in Medicaid). Given the Republican domination of the House, these cuts passed the House, but were opposed by Clinton. It became clear that year that Gingrich was willing to shut down the government if Clinton opposed the cuts. Government shutdowns occurred, first in mid-November and then again later in December after a temporary spending bill expired. One major aspect of the budget disagreement involved cuts in Medicare and Medicaid, along with other domestic programs. Eventually the government reopened and only modest cuts occurred in Medicare and Medicaid.

By the election year of 1996, everyone wanted a more successful session of Congress, and some minor reforms were passed in the health area, such as consolidation of programs that provided primary healthcare centers in certain communities and some healthcare for the homeless. Two more important reforms were added dealing with mental health and HMO care, as well as the passage of the Health Insurance Portability and Accountability Act of 1996, an act with some important healthcare reforms. The mental health provision may be more important as a reminder of the importance of mental health than in its immediate changes in the healthcare delivery system. The mental health provision requires that annual and lifetime caps on mental health benefits be at parity with those for physical illnesses. Some plans have had lifetime maximums of $50,000 for mental illness versus $1 million lifetime caps for physical illness. One limitation on the mental health provision is that it does not apply to small businesses with fewer than fifty employees.

The HMO provision in the Health Insurance Portability and Accountability Act was linked to maternity care and was a clear reaction to the growth of HMOs. As a cost-cutting technique, some managed care companies had put into effect policies that forced mothers to leave hospitals with their newborns fairly quickly, generally within twenty-four hours but in a few instances as soon as ten hours after a normal vaginal birth. By the time the federal law was enacted, thirty states had already enacted provisions similar to the new federal ones that require HMOs to allow mothers to stay in the hospital up to forty-eight hours after a normal vaginal delivery and up to ninety-six hours after a cesarean delivery. Thus, while the new law may not change the actual care available to many people, it sends an important message to HMOs that, given their growth, enrollees may be so concerned that they not only generate state restrictions, but even federal restrictions.

The main portions of the Health Insurance Portability and Accountability Act involve ending the hesitation of some people to take new jobs because of loss of health insurance due to the reimposition of preexisting clauses for serious health problems. The bill specifically prohibits employers who offer health coverage from limiting or denying coverage to individuals covered under a group health plan for more than twelve months for a medical condition that was diagnosed or treated in the previous six months. Once the twelve-month limit passes, no new preexisting limit may ever be imposed on people who maintain coverage with no more than a sixty-three-day gap, even if they change jobs or health plans. The legislation also prohibits employers from excluding an employee or dependent from coverage because their specific costs are too high. The legislation guarantees renewability of health coverage to employers and individuals except in the case of fraud or misrepresentation by an employer. The legislation also provides for medical savings accounts as an option for small businesses and the self-employed. This is important reform legislation and addresses several of the most important problems for employed individuals with health insurance.

The most important health-related piece of legislation under Clinton dealt with access-to-care issues. In fall 1997 Congress passed the new joint federal-state Children's Health Insurance Program (CHIP) as part of the Balanced Budget Act of 1997. This act initially made available $24 billion in funds to states over the five years from 1998 forward to help provide health insurance to children. This program was particularly aimed at children of the working poor, which often includes parents who are in the labor force but who work for an employer that does not provide healthcare insurance. The CHIP is having some success in improving the insurance levels of children. By 1999, 86 percent of children had health coverage, a small increase from 85 percent in 1998, and leading to the lowest rates of no insurance coverage for children since 1993. By 1999, 23 percent of children were covered by public programs such as Medicaid and the CHIP, as compared with only 11 percent in 1987, before the CHIP and some of the Medicaid expansions (Federal Interagency Forum Focus on Child and Family Statistics 2001).

Healthcare reform was not a major focus of the George W. Bush campaign, but some aspects of healthcare reform were discussed, especially a patients' rights bill and prescription-drug coverage for Medicare recipients. In summer 2001 many experts expected some action during the next congressional session on those issues, so that the Republicans would be able to point to some policy successes for the 2002 elections in November of that year. Instead, the terrorist attacks of September 11, 2001, occurred. Little domestic legislation passed in 2002, and the focus of the administration was on foreign-policy concerns, terrorism, the declining economy that was partially a result of the attacks, and scandals in the business community. The focus of the administration has continued to be on foreign policy, with the war against Iraq taking major attention in the first half of 2003 and issues with the reconstruction of Iraq continuing to be a major issue in the second half of 2003. The presence of a Republican majority in the Senate and a new leader of the Republicans, William Frist, who is a physician, has helped to focus some attention on healthcare issues in the second half of 2003. Although there is growing concern about the rising costs of health insurance, the future of reform in this area may come later, in 2004. The major health-related effort in the second half of 2003 was the passage of a Medicare reform bill. Though bitterly opposed by many Democrats and some Republicans, the legislation did pass at the end of November 2003. Although the measure has been publicized as providing drug coverage for the elderly, initially the plan will make available some prescription-drug cards in spring 2004. By 2006, seniors will be able to join privately administered drug plans for about $35 a month, and receive 75 percent of drug costs up to $2,250 after a $250 copayment. One reason for the opposition to the bill is that it also creates means testing for wealthier elderly persons beginning in 2007, so that higher-income elderly persons will pay more for Medicare benefits, and encourages the elderly to enter managed care plans. In addition, in 2010, Medicare would test competition between private health plans and the government in six metropolitan areas. Many liberals believe these two aspects of the bill will undermine the strength of the government program and could be a first step to the dismantling of Medicare. Also, over time, the commitment of the middle-class elderly to the program may diminish overall support if income ranges for the extra charges are not changed. The bill also provides substantial funding increases for some doctor and hospital services, and does nothing to control the costs of drugs. In the long run, this could lead to even greater concerns about rising healthcare costs in future years.

References

Andersen, Ronald M., and Pamela L. Davidson. 1996. Measuring Access and Trends. In *Changing the U.S. Health Care Delivery System*, edited by Ronald M. Andersen, Thomas H. Rice, and Gerald F. Kominski. San Francisco: Jossey-Bass Publishers.

Blendon, Robert J., Mollyann Brodie, and John Benson. 1995. What Happened to Americans' Support for the Clinton Health Plan? *Health Affairs* 14: 7–23.

DesHarnais, S., E. Kobrinski, and J. Chesney. 1987. The Early Effects of the PPS on Inpatient Utilization and the Quality of Care. *Inquiry* 24: 7–16.

Edwards, W. O., and C. R. Fisher. 1989. Medicare Physician and Hospital Utilization and Expenditure Trends. *Health Care Financing Review* 11: 111–116.

Federal Interagency Forum Focus on Child and Family Statistics. 2001. America's Children: Key National Indicators of Well-Being. Washington, DC: U.S. Government Printing Office.

Gay, G., J. J. Kronenfeld, S. Baker, and R. Amidon. 1989. An Appraisal of Organizational Response to Fiscally Constraining Regulation. *Journal of Health and Social Behavior* 30: 41–55.

Heclo, Hugh. 1995. The Clinton Health Plan: Historical Perspectives. *Health Affairs* 14: 86–98.

Himmelfarb, Richard. 1995. *Catastrophic Politics: The Rise and Fall of the Medicare Catastrophic Coverage Act of 1988*. University Park: Pennsylvania State University Press.

Hsiao, W. C., D. B. Yntema, P. Braun, and E. Becker. 1988. Resource Based Relative Values: An Overview. *Journal of the American Medical Association* 260: 2347–2353.

———. 1990. Refinement and Expansion of the Harvard RBRVS. *American Journal of Public Health* 80: 799–803.

Johnson, Haynes, and David S. Broder. 1996. *The System: The American Way of Politics at the Breaking Point*. Boston: Little, Brown.

Kingdon, John W. 1984. *Agendas, Alternatives and Public Policies*. Boston: Little, Brown.

Koch, A. L. 1988. Financing Health Systems. In *Introduction to Health Services*, 3rd ed., edited by Stephen J. Williams and Paul R. Torrens. New York: John Wiley and Sons.

Kronenfeld, Jennie Jacobs. 1997. *The Changing Federal Role in U.S. Health Care Policy*. Westport, CT: Praeger.

Lee, Phillip R., and A. E. Benjamin. 1993. Health Policy and the Politics of Health Care. In *Introduction to Health Services*, 4th ed., edited by Stephen J. Williams and Paul R. Torrens. Albany, NY: Delmar Publishers.

McIlrath, S. 1991a. HCFA Issues Final RBRVS Rules. *American Medical News* (December): 1, 26–47.

———. 1991b. RBRVS Launch Could Be Difficult. *American Medical News* (December): 1, 37.

Quadagno, Jill. 2002. *Aging and the Life Course: An Introduction to Social Gerontology*. 2nd ed. New York: McGraw Hill.

The Robert Wood Johnson Foundation. 1987. *Access to Health Care in the United States: Results of a 1986 Survey*. Special Report Number 2. Princeton, NJ: Robert Wood Johnson Foundation.

Skopcol, Theda. 1992. *Protecting Soldiers and Mothers: The Political Origins of Social Policy in the United States*. Cambridge, MA: Harvard University Press.

———. 1995. The Rise and Resounding Demise of the Clinton Plan. *Health Affairs* 14: 66–85.

Starr, Paul. 1982. *The Social Transformation of American Medicine: The Rise of a Sovereign Profession and the Making of a Vast Industry*. New York: Basic Books.

———. 1994. *The Logic of Healthcare Reform*. New York: Penguin Books.

Strickland, Stephen. 1978. *Research and the Health of Americans: Improving the Public Policy Process*. Lexington, MA: Lexington Books.

Wallace, Helen, Edward M. Gold, and Allan C. Oglesby. 1982. *Maternal and Child Health Practices: Problems, Resources and Methods of Delivery*. 2nd ed. New York: John Wiley and Sons.

Wiley, M. M. 1992. Hospital Financing Reform and Case-Mix Measurement: An International Review. *Health Care Financing Review* 13: 119–135.

Williams, Stephen J., and Paul R. Torrens. 1993. Influencing, Regulating and Monitoring the Health Care System. In *Introduction to Health Services*, 4th ed., edited by Stephen J. Williams and Paul R. Torrens. Albany, NY: Delmar Publishers.

Yankelovich, Daniel. 1995. The Debate That Wasn't: The Public and the Clinton Plan. *Health Affairs* 14: 7–23.

3

Chronology

1798 Merchant Marine Services Act (Act for the Relief of Sick and Disabled Seamen) of 1798 is the first federal act with any important health provisions. It provides health services to U.S. seamen by taxing the employers of merchant seamen. It funds the arrangements for their healthcare through the Marine Hospital Service.

1800 Legislation authorizes federal officials to cooperate with state and local officials to enforce quarantine laws.

Early 1800s The Merchant Marine Hospitals is established in major seaports of the United States, as authorized by the 1798 legislation, to deal with the healthcare needs of people in the merchant marine lines of work.

1862 The Morrill Act focuses on granting federal lands to each state and allowing the profits of those lands to be used for support of public institutions of higher education. These institutions become the land-grant colleges and host many programs in nursing and nutrition, and later, in medicine.

President Lincoln appoints a chemist, Charles M. Wetherill, to serve in the new Department of Agriculture. This is the beginning of the Bureau of Chemistry, forerunner to the Food and Drug Administration (FDA).

1870   The Marine Hospitals Services Act of 1870 provides a national agency with central headquarters to oversee Merchant Marine Hospitals and staffing. These hospitals had already been in existence, but the national agency with a central headquarters to deal with them is new.

1878   The Federal Quarantine Act of 1878 and amendments give the Marine Services Hospitals the authority to develop quarantine laws for ports that lack state or local regulation. Because immigration expands during this time frame, the act becomes important legislation that later expands to give the service full responsibility for foreign and interstate commerce.

1882   The first general immigration law includes provisions to exclude immigrants for medical reasons. To enforce this law, federal inspectors and doctors have to be allowed on board ships to check for diseases.

1887   The federal government opens a one-room laboratory on Staten Island for research on disease, thereby planting the seed that is to ultimately grow into the National Institutes of Health (NIH).

1899   The Commission Corps Act of 1899 and the amendments thereto allow the hiring of physicians and other health personnel to provide public health services.

1901   The U.S. Health Service Hygienic Laboratory is established.

1902   The Public Health and Marine Service Act of 1902 clarifies some federal health functions by renaming the Marine Hospital Service the Public Health and Marine Services. In addition, this act creates a system of communications among state, territorial, and federal health officials. The surgeon general, the administrative head of the Public Health Service (PHS), is authorized to have an annual meeting of state and territorial health officers to discuss major health policy issues and concerns of the day.

The Biologics Control Act of 1902 gives the PHS the responsibility to license and regulate biologically de-rived health products.

1906 The Pure Food and Drug Act of 1906 (Wiley Act) al-lows the Bureau of Chemistry in the Department of Agriculture to prohibit shipment of impure foods and drugs across state lines. By giving this authority to the Bureau of Chemistry, the act makes it possible for the bureau to regulate drug products and later to cre-ate specialized categories of drugs such as controlled substances in the case of narcotics and opium-derived drugs.

1912 President Theodore Roosevelt's first White House Conference urges creation of a Children's Bureau to combat exploitation of children. The conference deals with many aspects of the lives of children, including health-related concerns.

1917 The Vocational Educational Act of 1917 (Smith-Hughes Act) provides funds to establish early li-censed practical nursing (LPN) programs.

1920 The Snyder Act of 1920 is the first federal legislation to deal with healthcare for Native Americans. The act provides general assistance and directs the Bureau of Indian Affairs to direct, supervise, and expend monies for the benefit, care, and assistance of Native Americans throughout the United States, setting up the beginnings of what later became the Indian Health Service (IHS).

1921 The Maternity and Infancy Act of 1921 (Sheppard-Towner Act) provides grants to states to plan mater-nal and child health services. Although the law is al-lowed to lapse in 1929, it is very important because the mechanism of providing grants to states is new within the health area, and thus the legislation serves as a prototype for federal grants-in-aid to the states in the area of health.

1924   The Veterans Act of 1924 codifies and extends the role of the federal government in the provision of health-care services to veterans.

1930   The Ransdell Act of 1930 creates the National Institute of Health from the U.S. Health Service Hygienic Laboratory and sets in place the growth of federally funded health research through the different institutes of health that are now part of the modern National Institutes of Health (NIH).

     The Veterans' Administration is created as an independent U.S. government agency.

1932   The Committee on the Costs of Medical Care report is published and raises concerns about the costs of medical care at this time and the numbers of people who are effectively denied access to healthcare services due to the costs and their limited incomes.

1935   The Social Security Act of 1935, including Title V of the act, provides for a system of old-age pensions and other old-age benefits. This landmark legislation passes partially as a reaction to the Great Depression. In addition to the overall establishment of the old-age pension system, Title V includes grants to states for maternal, child health, and child welfare services, and for services to crippled children. The act also provides incentives for the establishment of state unemployment funds. Title VI authorizes annual federal grants to states for investigation of the problems of disease and sanitation, leading to the creation of new local health departments and overall significantly increasing federal assistance for state and local public health programs.

1937   The Social Security Act is expanded to include benefits for spouses and widows.

     An additional nationally funded health research institute is created, the National Cancer Institute, which later also becomes part of the National Institutes of Health (NIH).

1938   The Federal Food, Drug and Cosmetic Act of 1938 and the amendments thereto regulate for safety the market entry of new drug, cosmetic, and therapeutic products by extending the federal authority to ban new drugs from the market until they are approved by the Food and Drug Administration (FDA).

The Venereal Disease Control Act of 1938 (LaFollette-Bulwinkle Act) coordinates state efforts to combat syphilis and gonorrhea by providing grants-in-aid to the states to support their investigation and control of venereal disease.

1939   The Reorganization Act of 1939 plays a major role in the reorganization of many health-related functions in the federal government. The act transfers the Public Health Service (PHS) from the Treasury Department to the new Federal Security Agency (FSA). This is changed again in 1953 with the creation of the Department of Health, Education and Welfare (DHEW) and in 1980 with the creation of the Department of Health and Human Services (DHHS).

1944   The Public Health Service Act of 1944, a multipart act, makes many changes in the role of the federal government in public health services. The act specifies a role for the U.S. Public Health Service (PHS) in working with state and local health departments. It also revises and consolidates into one place all existing legislation pertaining to the PHS, and provides for the organization, staffing, and functions and activities of the PHS. The act also incorporates the provisions of the Biologics Control Act as a PHS responsibility, including allowing use of quarantines and inspections for the control of communicable diseases. Services are extended to inmates of penal and correctional institutions. The act is subsequently used as a vehicle, through amendments to the legislation, for a number of important federal grant-in-aid programs.

1945   The McCarran-Fergurson Act of 1945 exempts the business of insurance from federal antitrust legislation

1945 *(cont.)*	(such as the Sherman Antitrust Act of 1890 and the Clayton Act of 1914). This act provides instead that insurance is to be regulated by state law, and the act does not involve acts of boycott, coercion, or intimidation as the reason why insurance, including health insurance, is exempted.
1946	The U.S. National Health Policy Hospital Survey and Construction Act of 1946 (Hill-Burton Amendments to the Public Health Service Act [PHS]) provides grants to states to inventory and survey existing hospital and public healthcare facilities in each state and to plan for new ones. The new act authorizes grants to both survey existing facilities and plan construction of new facilities, as well as grants to assist in such construction. As part of this initiation of a process of planning about health facilities, the act requires the establishment of state planning agencies and submission of a state plan for the construction of hospital facilities to receive the federal funds.
	The National Mental Health Act of 1946 (an amendment to the PHS of 1944) authorizes federal support for mental health research and treatment programs. Included in the federal support is the authorization of grants-in-aid to the states for mental health activities. The act transforms the Division of Mental Health in the PHS into the National Institute of Mental Health.
1948	The National Health Act of 1948 expands the capacity of the National Institute of Health by making it the National Institutes of Health (NIH) and creating a second categorical institute, the National Heart Institute.
1953	The Federal Security Agency is renamed and given department status as the Department of Health, Education and Welfare (DHEW).
1954	Medical Facilities Survey and Construction Act of 1954. These amendments to the U.S. National Health

Policy Hospital Survey and Construction Act of 1946 (the Hill-Burton Act) greatly expand the program's scope by authorizing grants for surveys and construction of diagnostic and treatment centers, including hospital outpatient departments, chronic disease hospitals, rehabilitation facilities, and nursing homes.

1956   The Health Amendments Act of 1956, which amends the basic Public Health Service Act of 1944, adds special projects dealing with problems of state mental hospitals. The act also authorizes federal assistance for the education and training of health personnel, including traineeships for public health personnel and for the advanced training of nurses.

The Dependents Medical Care Act of 1956 establishes the Civilian Health and Medical Program of the Uniformed Services (CHAMPUS) for the dependents of military personnel.

1958   The Food Additives Amendment of 1958 amends the Federal Food, Drug and Cosmetic Act of 1938 to require premarketing clearance from the Food and Drug Administration (FDA) for new food additives. This new act includes the Delaney clause, named after Representative James Delaney, stating that no additive shall be deemed to be safe if it is found to induce cancer when ingested by human or animal.

1959   The Federal Employees Health Benefit Act of 1959 permits Blue Cross to negotiate a contract with the Civil Service Commission to provide health insurance coverage for federal employees.

1960   The Social Security Amendments of 1960 (Kerr-Mills Act) amend the Social Security Act to establish a program of medical assistance for the aged. Through this program, the act also provides aid to the states for payments for medical care for "medically indigent" persons who are sixty-five years of age or older. The participation by states is optional, with only twenty-five states participating. The Kerr-Mills program is

1960 *(cont.)*	the forerunner of the Medicaid program established in 1965.
1961	Community Health Services and Facilities Act of 1961. Although this act is passed as a separate statute, the act mostly amends the U.S. National Health Policy Hospital Survey and Construction Act of 1946 (the Hill-Burton Act of 1946) by increasing the amount of funds available for nursing-home construction and by extending the research and demonstration grant program to other medical facilities.
1962	The Health Services for Agricultural Migratory Workers Act of 1962 (an amendment to the Public Health Service Act of 1944) establishes a program of federal grants for family clinics and other health services for migrant workers and their families.
	The Drug Amendments of 1962 (Kefauver-Harris Amendments) modify the Federal Food, Drug and Cosmetic Act of 1938 to significantly strengthen the provisions related to the regulation of therapeutic drugs. They also require improved manufacturing processes and procedures and evidence to assure that new drugs proposed for marketing are effective as well as safe. The amendments follow widespread negative publicity about the serious negative side effects of the drug thalidomide and reflect the concerns of Americans about ensuring the safety of new drugs.
1963	Maternal and Child Health and Mental Retardation Planning Amendments; Amendments to Title V of the Social Security Act in 1963, 1965, and 1967. These amendments modify the basic Social Security Act to assist states and communities in preventing and combating mental retardation through expansion and improvement of the maternal, child, and crippled children's programs. They also add special project grants for maternity and infant care for low-income mothers and infants and add special project grants for child dental services.

The Health Professions Education Assistance Act of 1963 (an amendment to the Public Health Service Act) provides construction grants for facilities that train physicians, nurses, dentists, podiatrists, pharmacists, and public health personnel. The act also provides for student-loan funds and scholarship funds to schools of medicine and osteopathy. It also includes construction grants that are contingent upon schools increasing their first-year enrollments. Later amendments extend loan funds to a variety of health and allied health professions.

1964   The first Surgeon General's Report on Smoking and Health is released, and thus begins the growing public recognition of the negative health effects of smoking.

The Nurse Training Act of 1964 provides schools of nursing with support to permit them to increase enrollments and improve their physical facilities.

1965   The Health Professions Educational Assistance Amendments of 1965 (which amend the 1963 act) authorize basic improvement (institutional grants), special improvement grants, and scholarship grants to schools of medicine, dentistry, osteopathy, optometry, and podiatry. The amendments also authorize scholarship grants to schools of pharmacy, expand the student-loan program, and include a provision through which 50 percent of a professional student's loan can be forgiven in exchange for practice in a designated shortage area.

Health Insurance for the Aged of 1965—Title XVIII of the Social Security Act (Medicare) and amendments. Through these amendments, a program of national health insurance for elderly Social Security recipients is established. Part A provides basic protection against the costs of hospitalization and selected posthospital services. Part B is a voluntary program financed by premium payments from enrollees with matching federal revenues and provides supplemental medical insurance benefits. In later

1965
(cont.)
years, additional amendments extend coverage to patients who receive cash payments under the disability provisions of the Social Security Act and thus provide health insurance for the aged with federal funds. Because of the use of federal funds, this act also becomes the mechanism for later federal regulations dealing with quality assurance, institutional minimum standards, utilization review, and cost controls.

Grants to the States for Medical Assistance Programs of 1965—Title XIX of the Social Security Act (Medicaid) and amendments. These amendments create a federal-state matching program with voluntary state participation to partially replace the Kerr-Mills program. These amendments provide a federally supported (with state matching funds) program that provides some healthcare services for the categorically poor receiving welfare payments. Participating states have to provide five basic services: inpatient and outpatient, other laboratory and X-ray, physician, and skilled nursing-home services. In addition, states can include a number of other optional services. Over time, the required and optional services change with amendments, as does the eligibility of various groups of the poor. Although federal categorical welfare recipients are eligible from the beginning, by option, states can include medically needy with incomes too high for cash federal welfare payments through the provision of health services for low-income federal public-assistance recipients and the medically needy. Eventually, the linkage with receipt of welfare benefits is removed, but the program remains a means-tested one with income eligibility rules. As with Medicare, the program becomes a mechanism for federal regulation of quality assurance, institutional minimum standards, utilization review, and cost controls in healthcare.

The Older Americans Act of 1965 establishes an Administration on Aging to administer, through state agencies, programs for the elderly. There are ten specific covered objectives for the elderly, including several relating to health.

1966 The Comprehensive Health Planning and Public Health Service Amendments of 1966 (Partnership for Health) provide for state and local planning for health services facilities through A (state level) and B (community level) agencies. Block grants are provided to state health departments for discretionary purposes. The act seeks to create comprehensive planning for health facilities, services, and personnel within the framework of a federal-state-local partnership. Section 314a authorizes grants to states for the development of comprehensive state health planning while Section 314b authorizes grants to public or nonprofit organizations for developing comprehensive regional, metropolitan area, or other local area plans.

1967 Mental Health Amendments of 1967 and Mental Retardation Amendments to the Mental Retardation Facilities and Community Mental Health Centers Construction Act of 1960. These amendments extend construction grants to community mental health centers to cover acquisition of existing buildings. The act also extends the program of construction grants for university-affiliated and community-based facilities for the mentally retarded.

The Social Security Amendments of 1967 are the first of many modifications to the Medicare and Medicaid programs established first by the Social Security Amendments of 1960. These amendments provide expanded coverage for durable medical equipment for use in the home, podiatrist services, and outpatient physical therapy, and add sixty days of coverage for inpatient hospital care over and above the original coverage for up to ninety days during any spell of illness. Some payment rules are also modified, generally in favor of providers of care. New conditions are provided that have to be met by nursing homes wanting to participate in the Medicare and Medicaid programs as part of a quality-control mechanism.

1970   The Comprehensive Drug Abuse and Prevention and Control Act of 1970 provides for special project grants for drug abuse and drug dependence treatment programs and programs related to drug education.

The Poison Prevention and Packaging Act of 1970 requires that most drugs be dispensed in containers designed to be difficult for children to open.

The Comprehensive Alcohol Abuse and Alcoholism Prevention, Treatment, and Rehabilitation Act of 1970 establishes the National Institute of Alcohol Abuse and Alcoholism. The act also provides a separate statutory base for programs and activities relating to alcohol abuse and alcoholism, including a program of aid to states and localities in their efforts to combat alcohol abuse and alcoholism.

The Communicable Disease Control Amendments of 1970 (amendments to the Public Health Service Act of 1944) reestablish categorical grant programs to control communicable diseases such as tuberculosis, venereal disease, measles, and rubella. They also rename the CDC the Centers for Disease Control and broadens its concern beyond the communicable diseases to other preventable conditions such as malnutrition, certain chronic health problems, and accidental injuries.

1971   The Comprehensive Health Manpower Training Act of 1971 (a Public Health Service Act amendment) is a complex series of amendments that replace institutional grants with a new system of capitation grants in which health professions schools receive fixed sums of money for each student enrolled contingent on increasing first-year enrollments. The act also creates project grants and financial-distress grants and revises loan and scholarship provisions so that 85 percent of education loans to a student can be canceled by health professionals who practice in a designated shortage area. The legislation also establishes the National Health Manpower Clearinghouse and directs the Secretary of the Department of Health, Education and Welfare (DHEW, now the Department of Health and Human Services [DHHS]) to make every effort to provide to counties without physicians at least one National Health Service Corps physician.

The National Cancer Act is signed into law.

1972   Social Security Amendments of 1972 to the Social Security Act of 1935 and the Medicare and Medicaid Amendments of 1965. These amendments make significant changes in the Medicare program to try to control growing costs. One of the ways to control costs is through the establishment of Professional Standards Review Organizations (PSROs) that are to monitor both the quality of services provided to Medicare beneficiaries as well as the medical necessity for the services. Payment for capital expenditures that have been disapproved by state or local planning agencies is limited. The act also authorizes a program of grants and contracts to conduct experiments to achieve increased efficiency and economy in the provision of health services and also increases access to services for certain groups of people (which raises the costs of the program). For the first time, people who are eligible for cash benefits under the disability provision of the Social Security Act for at least twenty-four months are made eligible for medical benefits under the program. Also, persons insured under Social Security and their dependents who require hemodialysis or renal transplantation are defined as disabled for the purpose of having them covered under the Medicare program for the costs of treating their end-stage renal disease (ESRD).

1973   The Health Maintenance Organization Act of 1973 (an amendment to the Public Health Service Act) and amendments in 1976, 1978, and 1981 are aimed at encouraging the development of health maintenance organizations (HMOs). The act specifies the basic medical services that an HMO has to provide to be eligible for federal funding, including specified

1973
(cont.)
requirements for fiscal responsibility for broad population enrollment and a policy-making board. As a way to encourage enrollment in HMOs, it is mandated that every employer of twenty-five or more persons offer an HMO option. Later amendments mitigate the stringency of the original requirements for HMO service provision to be eligible for federal funding.

1974
The National Health Planning and Resources Development Act of 1974 (an amendment to the Public Health Service Act PL-93-641) adds two new titles, XV and XVI, to the Public Health Service Act and substantially replaces the programs established under Sections 314a and 314b of the Comprehensive Health Planning and Public Health Service Amendments of 1966, as well as some of the provisions of the U.S. National Health Policy Hospital Survey and Construction Act of 1946 (the Hill-Burton Act), by creating a system of local and state planning agencies supported through federal funds. This includes the designation of State Health Planning and Development Agencies (SHPDAs) and State Health Coordinating Councils (SHCCs), along with creating a network of local Health Systems Agencies (HSAs) to improve the health of area residents. The HSAs are also supposed to increase accessibility, acceptability, continuity, and quality of health services and to play a role in the restraining of health cost increases by preventing duplication of healthcare services and facilities. As part of the control over too much duplication of services, the law permits the states to establish certificate-of-need (CON) programs to conduct reviews and make recommendations about new healthcare facilities and services. States can also regulate funds for new capital expenditures and for renovations for health institutions, and provide assistance for modernization or construction of inpatient and outpatient facilities. Although this is a major piece of legislation that for over a decade creates a system of local- and state-based planning in terms of healthcare facilities, it is repealed by Congress in

1986, leaving the responsibility for CON programs entirely in the hands of states.

1976   The Medical Devices Amendment of 1976 (an amendment to the Federal Food, Drug and Cosmetic Act of 1948) strengthens the regulation of medical devices partially as a reaction to concerns over the Dalkon Shield intrauterine device.

1977   The Health Care Financing Administration is created to manage Medicare and Medicaid separately from the Social Security Administration.

The Health Maintenance Organization Amendments of 1977 (amending the 1973 Health Maintenance Organization Act) ease the requirements that have to be met for a Health Maintenance Organization (HMO) to be federally qualified and require that an HMO has to be federally qualified to receive Medicare and Medicaid funds.

The Indian Health Care Improvement Act of 1977 deals with filling gaps in the delivery of healthcare services to Native Americans, mostly through the Indian Health Service (IHS).

The Rural Health Care Services Amendments of 1977 (amendments to the Medicare and Medicaid legislation of 1965) modify the categories of practitioners that can provide services under these programs. Rural health clinics that do not routinely have physicians on site can be reimbursed for services provided by nurse practitioners if they meet certain requirements. The amendments also authorize demonstration projects with these practitioners for underserved urban areas.

The Medicare and Medicaid Antifraud and Abuse Amendments of 1977 (amendments to the Medicare and Medicaid legislation of 1965) are passed as part of an effort to try to reduce fraud and abuse in the programs as a means to help contain costs. The

1977
(cont.)

amendments strengthen criminal and civil penalties for fraud and abuse, modify the operation of Professional Standards Review Organizations (PSROs), and require uniform reporting systems and formats for hospitals and certain other healthcare organizations participating in Medicare and Medicaid.

1980

The Omnibus Budget Reconciliation Act (OBRA) of 1980 begins a new trend of omnibus legislation covering many aspects of health and other policy areas being passed as part of the budget reconciliation process. The act is contained as part of Title IX of the Medicare and Medicaid Amendments of 1980. This act makes extensive modifications in the Medicare and Medicaid program aimed at dealing with the growing costs of the programs. For Medicare, examples of some of the changes include the removal of the 100-visits-per-year limitation on home health services, the requirement of a deductible for home care visits under part B, the granting of permission to small rural hospitals to use swing beds (which alternate between acute or long-term care beds as the need occurs), and the authorizing of demonstration programs of swing beds in large urban hospitals. The most important change for Medicaid is requiring the program to pay for the services that the states have authorized nurse-midwives to perform.

1981

Omnibus Budget Reconciliation Act (OBRA) of 1981 (in Title XXI, Subtitles A, B, and C as further amendments to the Medicare and Medicaid programs). This legislation also includes extensive changes to the Medicare and Medicaid programs with forty-six sections, including eliminating the coverage of alcohol detoxification facilities, removing occupational therapy as a basis for entitlement for home health services, and increasing the part B deductible. In addition, the amendments replace twenty categorical programs in areas of prevention, alcohol and drug abuse, mental health, primary care, and some areas of maternal and child health with block grants in four of the major areas listed above. In addition, the legisla-

tion reduces funds by 25 percent in the process of replacing categorical programs with block grants. In the
preventive-programs area, the act consolidates separate programs such as rodent control, fluoridation,
hypertension control, and rape crisis centers into one
block grant distributed among the states by a formula
based on population and other factors. In the mental
health area, the act combines the existing programs
under the Community Mental Health Centers Act, the
Mental Health Systems Act, the Comprehensive Alcohol Abuse and Alcoholism Prevention, Treatment,
and Rehabilitation Act, and the Drug Abuse and Prevention, Treatment and Rehabilitation Act. For legislation relating to primary care, the block grant replaces the Community Health Centers, and in the
Maternal and Child Health block grant consolidates
seven categorical programs from Title V of the Social
Security Act and the Public Health Service Act, including maternal health and crippled children's programs, Sudden Infant Death Syndrome (SIDS), genetic disease services, hemophilia treatment, Social
Security Insurance (SSI) payments to disabled children, and lead-based poisoning programs.

Acquired Immune Deficiency Syndrome (AIDS) is
identified. In 1984, the human immunodeficiency
virus (HIV) is identified by the Public Health Service
and French scientists. In 1985, a blood test to detect
HIV is licensed.

1982   The Tax Equity and Fiscal Responsibility Act (TEFRA)
of 1982 makes important changes in the Medicare and
Medicaid programs and in some other health-related
programs. It replaces Professional Standards Review
Organizations (PSROs) that had been established by
the Social Security Amendments of 1972 and elimi-
nates requirements for local Health Systems Agencies
(HSAs), cuts their funding, and increases gubernator-
ial discretion concerning their future role. The act also
replaces PSROs with Professional Review Organizations (PROs) and makes their use in hospitals optional
for patients covered under government programs. The

1982 (cont.)	act makes some changes in reimbursement and methodology for both Medicare and Medicaid. For Medicare, the act makes extensive changes in reimbursement methodologies for hospital-related services under Medicare and begins a shift to case mix (diagnosis-related groups [DRGs]) for reimbursements for most acute-care hospitals. In addition, the act eliminates nursing salary cost differentials and private-room subsidies, eliminates the lesser-of-cost-or-charge provision, and makes reimbursement changes for health maintenance organizations (HMOs). For Medicaid, the act tightens regulations on acceptable error rates and overpayments, and makes a number of changes in payment methodology. It also adds coverage for hospice services to Medicare benefits and reduces Medicaid funding for states, but allows a partial gain back for improved program administration, including fraud detection and error-rate reduction. Changes in manpower and personnel policy also occur through this act, which eliminates capitation payments for nursing and medical schools and reduces capitation payments for selected other health professional schools and also greatly reduces funding for new entrants into the National Health Service Corps.
1983	The Social Security Amendments of 1983 include a major landmark in the Medicare program. This legislation amends the basic rules of the Medicare program to be a prospective payment system for hospital care by basing payments to hospitals on predetermined rates per discharge for diagnosis-related groups (DRGs) as contrasted to the earlier cost-based system of reimbursement that had been used since the initial passage of the Medicare program. In addition, the act authorizes a study of physician-payment reform options.
1984	The Deficit Reduction Act (DEFRA) of 1984 temporarily freezes increases in physician payment under Medicare and places a specific limit on the rate of increase in the diagnosis-related group (DRG) payment

rates in the following two years. It also establishes the Medicare Participating Physician and Supplier Program (PAR) that creates two classes of physicians in regard to their relationships to the Medicare program and outlines different reimbursement approaches for them depending upon whether one was classified as "participating" or "nonparticipating." Additionally, the act mandates that the Office of Technology Assessment study alternative means of paying for physicians' services to guide reform of Medicare.

The National Organ Transplant Act is signed into law.

1985   The Consolidated Omnibus Budget Reconciliation Act of 1985 (COBRA 1985) especially impacts the Medicare program by an adjustment in the disproportionate share payments made to hospitals that serve many poor patients. In addition, hospice care is made a permanent part of Medicare and made available to states also for Medicaid. The act freezes Medicare Prospective Payment System (PPS) payment rates for part of a year and provides modified hospital indirect rates for medical education. The act also establishes the Physician Payment Review Commission (PPRC) to aid Congress on physician-payment policies and requires that employers continue health insurance for employees and their dependents who would otherwise lose their eligibility due to reduced hours or termination of employment.

1986   The Omnibus Budget Reconciliation Act of 1986 (OBRA 1986) alters the Prospective Payment System (PPS) payment rate for hospitals, reduces payment amounts for capital-related costs, and establishes further limits to balance billing by physicians by setting maximum-allowable charges for physicians who do not participate in the Participating Physician and Supplier Program (PAR).

The Omnibus Health Act of 1986 liberalizes coverage under the Medicaid program by using federal income up to the federal poverty line as a criterion. (The

1986
(cont.)

change allows states to offer all pregnant women and infants up to one year of coverage with a phase-in schedule up to five years of age.) The act also includes the National Childhood Vaccine Injury Act that establishes a federal vaccine-injury compensation program system. Another portion, the Health Care Quality Improvement Act, provides immunity from private damage lawsuits under federal or state law for a professional review action that follows standards set out in the legislation.

1987

The Omnibus Budget Reconciliation Act of 1987 (OBRA 1987) alters a number of aspects of both Medicare and Medicaid. For Medicare, the major changes are that the wage index used to calculate hospital payments is updated and capital-related costs are reduced by 12 percent for fiscal year 1988 and 15 percent for fiscal year 1989. For physician payment, fees for twelve overvalued procedures are reduced and higher fee increases are allowed for primary care than for specialized physician services. For Medicaid, states are required to cover eligible children up to age six with an option for up to age eight. In addition, the distinction between skilled nursing facilities and intermediate-care facilities is eliminated, and a number of provisions designed to enhance the quality of care in nursing homes are included.

1988

The National Organ Transplant Amendments of 1988 amend the National Organ Transplant Act of 1984 to extend the prohibition against the sale of human organs to the organs and body parts of human fetuses.

The Medicare Catastrophic Coverage Act (an amendment to the Medicare Act of 1965) provides the largest expansion of benefits since the creation of the program, including some added coverage for outpatient drugs and respite care. The act places a cap on out-of-pocket spending for copayment costs and covered services. The funding for the program is to come from increased premiums to all Medicare enrollees and an income-related supplemental premium. Once the act is passed and the elderly realize that many of the additional costs will impact the elderly the most, some groups of the elderly become upset. Because many elderly (especially the more affluent) already have some of these services, and because they realize that long-term care services are not going to be covered, there is dissension about the act, and it is repealed before provisions go into effect.

The McKinney Act is signed into law, providing healthcare to the homeless.

1989   The Omnibus Budget Reconciliation Act of 1989 (OBRA 1989) includes provisions for minor, predominantly technical changes in the Prospective Payment System (PPS). These include some coverage for mental health benefits and Pap smears and small adjustments in disproportionate-share rules. The major change is to begin the implementation of a resource-based relative value scale (RBRVS) for physician payment, phased in over a four-year period starting in 1992. Also, a new agency, the Agency for Health Care Policy and Research (AHCPR), is created to replace the National Center for Health Services Research and Technology Assessment (NCHSR). The focus of the new agency is to conduct and foster the conducting of studies of healthcare quality, effectiveness, and efficiency, including those conducted on outcomes of medical care treatment.

1990   The Americans with Disabilities Act (ADA) of 1990 provides a broad range of protections for the disabled, and thus combines former protections from the Civil Rights Act of 1964, the Rehabilitation Act of 1973, and the Civil Rights Restoration Act of 1988. The ADA legislation helps the disabled toward a goal of independence and self-support, and gives them greater rights in a variety of settings, such as schools and workplaces.

The Ryan White Comprehensive AIDS Resources Emergency Act of 1990 (an amendment to the Public

1990
(cont.)

Health Service Act of 1944) sets up special programs to distribute funds related to AIDS through grants. The act also creates mechanisms to involve the public in the process and creates mechanisms for planning and evaluation of the process.

The Omnibus Budget Reconciliation Act of 1990 (OBRA 1990) includes the Patient Self-Determination Act, a variety of minor changes in the Prospective Payment System (PPS), and other technical adjustments to payments for Medicare. The Patient Self-Determination Act requires healthcare institutions that participate in Medicare and Medicaid to provide all patients with written information on policies regarding self-determination and living wills, and to inquire whether patients have advance medical directives. The act also makes further adjustments in the PPS wage-index calculation and the capital-related payment reduction. As part of deficit reduction, the act includes a five-year deficit-reduction plan to reduce Medicare outlays by over $43 billion between fiscal years 1991 and 1995. Another important change is to require that all Medigap policies sold after July 1992 conform to one of ten standardized packages so that consumers can more easily compare coverage and costs from one insurance company to another.

The Human Genome Project is established.

1993

The National Institutes of Health Revitalization Act of 1993 provides for some structural and budgetary changes in the operation of the National Institutes of Health (NIH). This act includes guidelines for the conduct of research on transplantation of human fetal tissue and adds HIV infection to the list of excludable conditions covered by the Immigration and Nationality Act.

The Omnibus Budget Reconciliation Act of 1993 (OBRA 1993) puts into place a record five-year cut in Medicare funding and includes other changes in Medicare such as a provision to end return-on-equity

(ROE) payments for capital to proprietary skilled nursing facilities (SNFs). The act reduces the rate of increase of inpatient rates for care provided in hospices, cuts laboratory fees, and freezes payments for durable medical equipment, parenteral and enteral services, and orthotics and prosthetics.

The Childhood Immunization Act supports the provision of vaccines for children eligible for Medicaid, children without health insurance, and Native American children.

1994   The Social Security Act Amendments of 1994 make a number of technical and other changes in the Medicare program. These include a modified Maternal and Child Health block-grant program and modified income security, human resources, and related programs for Medicare. The amendments also adjust standardized amounts for wages and wage-related costs. The amendments also provide more coverage for psychologists, refine the geographic-cost-of-practice index for physician payment, limit extra billing of physicians, and require the creation of complete relative values for pediatric services as had been done earlier for other types of services. The amendments also modify durable medical equipment rules and set in place mammography certification requirements. The legislation also places an annual cap on Medicare payment for outpatient physical therapy and occupational therapy services and provides speech-language pathology and audiology services. In the maternal and child welfare area, the legislation increases the authorization and places more emphasis on protections for foster children, child welfare traineeships, and payments of state claims for foster care and adoption assistance. This act adds new enforcement procedures in child support programs along with other changes linked more closely to welfare than to medical services.

The Veterans Health Programs Extension Act of 1994 adds the treatment of sexual trauma and repeals the

1994
(cont.)
limitation on time to seek services for this issue. The act increases research relating to women veterans and increases authority to provide priority healthcare for veterans exposed to toxic substances.

Scientists supported by the National Institutes of Health (NIH) discover the genes responsible for many cases of hereditary colon cancer, inherited breast cancer, and the most common type of kidney cancer.

1995
The Social Security Administration becomes an independent agency on March 31.

1996
The Health Insurance Portability and Accountability Act of 1996 (also known as the Kennedy-Kassebaum Act) improves portability and continuity of health insurance coverage in group and individual markets when an individual loses a job. The act also promotes the use of medical savings accounts, improves access to long-term care services and coverage, and provides for changes in membership and duties of the national committee on vital and health statistics.

The Health Centers Consolidation Act of 1996 (an amendment to the Public Health Service Act of 1944 and its amendments) consolidates and more clearly defines health centers, primary care services, and medically underserved areas. Included as part of this legislation is the planning of grants and managed care loan guarantees. There are some special provisions for services to the homeless.

The Indian Health Care Improvement Technical Corrections Act of 1996 (amendment to the Indian Health Care Improvement Act of 1977) extends demonstration programs for direct billing of Medicare, Medicaid, and other third-party payers.

The Veterans Health Care Eligibility Reform Act of 1996 amends previous veterans' healthcare legislation so as to reform eligibility for healthcare provided by the Department of Veterans Affairs. The act also makes changes related to the provision of care as to the extent and amount provided in advance by authorization legislation, and, as part of this, outpatient care priorities separate from inpatient care priorities are deleted. Some major facility-construction projects for the department are allowed, as are improved administration of healthcare by the department. More care is provided for women veterans, including readjustment counseling and mental health care. Special studies on hospice care begin, along with special pay arrangements for physicians and dentists who enter residency training. There is also a provision for evaluation of the health status of spouses and children of Persian war veterans.

The Ryan White Care Act Amendments of 1996 (amendments to the Ryan White Comprehensive AIDS Resources Emergency Act of 1990) set new definitions of eligible areas and eligible population numbers, and make modifications in membership of the councils to aid in distribution of funds. Grievance procedures are modified for grant distribution, and some aspects of grant application and planning and evaluation are modified.

Welfare reform is enacted under the Personal Responsibility and Work Opportunity Reconciliation Act. This act modifies welfare and changes programs such as the Aid to Families with Dependent Children (AFDC) program to the Temporary Assistance to Needy Families (TANF) program. This legislation provides for limits on how long someone can remain on welfare and adds work requirements.

1997   The State Children's Health Insurance Program (CHIP) is established. This is passed as an addition to the Medicaid program, and states have to pass enabling legislation to participate. States can set this up as a part of Medicaid or as a separate program.

1998   The Initiative to Eliminate Racial and Ethnic Dispari-
        ties in Health is launched. This Clinton initiative com-
        mits the nation to the goal of eliminating disparities
        in various areas of health status by racial and ethnic
        minority status by 2010.

1999   The Ticket to Work and Work Incentives Improve-
        ment Act of 1999 is signed, making it possible for mil-
        lions of Americans with disabilities to join the work-
        force without fear of losing their Medicaid and
        Medicare coverage. It also modernizes the employ-
        ment services system for people with disabilities.

        Initiative on combating bioterrorism is launched.

2000   Human genome sequencing is published.

2001   The Centers for Medicare and Medicaid Services is
        created, replacing the Health Care Financing Admin-
        istration. Although this is mostly an administrative
        change, it does focus attention more clearly on how
        the Medicare program and how the federal aspects of
        the Medicaid program work.

4

People and Events

George W. Bush (July 6, 1946–)

George W. Bush is the forty-third president of the United States, having taken office on January 20, 2001, after the controversial election in 2000. Bush's healthcare agenda (http://www. whitehouse.gov/infocus/medicare/health-care/) is based upon patient choice within the current system. His proposal involves changes in current programs rather than a major reformulation of the system, as he does not support a single-payer, national healthcare system. Many critics do not feel that his proposals adequately address the crisis caused by rapidly rising healthcare costs.

Hillary Rodham Clinton (October 26, 1947–)

Hillary Rodham Clinton is the wife of Bill Clinton, the forty-second president of the United States. With a law degree from Yale, she was the first first lady to have her own career at the time her husband was elected as president. She served as a key policy advisor to her husband and led the failed effort in 1993 and 1994 to pass comprehensive reform of the U.S. healthcare system. This failure was largely the result of both Clintons' lack of experience in national politics. Much of the development of the plan was done without significant input from the key congressional leaders. Although there was a process of input that included industry leaders, health policy analysts, and government officials, this group was not able to reach a consensus about a proposal quickly enough to ensure the emergence of a strong-enough coalition to lead to its passage. For the rest of her husband's presidency, she adopted a somewhat lower profile, although her interests in politics remained strong. This was most clearly demonstrated by her decision to seek her first elective office by running for the U.S. Senate seat in New York. She succeeded in this effort and was elected to the U.S. Senate from New York in 2000.

William (Bill) Jefferson Clinton (August 19, 1946–)

William (Bill) Jefferson Clinton was the forty-second president of the United States, serving from 1993 to 2001. He was the first Democrat since Franklin Roosevelt to be elected to a second term. A major campaign promise in his first campaign in 1993 was to enact a major reform in the U.S. healthcare system that would ensure access to all while controlling costs. He appointed his wife, Hillary, to lead the effort to develop and enact a national healthcare proposal. This effort at developing a national healthcare system was unsuccessful (see the "Hillary Rodham Clinton" entry in this chapter). After this failure in 1994 and the subsequent loss of control of the House of Representatives to the Republican Party, Clinton declared the era of big government over and, instead, focused on incremental change in government programs including health-related programs. The subsequent healthcare reform programs passed included the Children's Health Insurance Program (CHIP). This program is focused upon provision of health insurance to children of the working poor and near poor, and it represents the largest expansion of direct government programs to provide health insurance coverage to Americans since the passage of Medicare and Medicaid in 1965.

Wilbur J. Cohen (June 10, 1913– May 17, 1987)

Wilbur J. Cohen had a long career in government services and in education. After graduating from the University of Wisconsin in 1934, he took the job as research assistant to Executive Director Witte of President Roosevelt's cabinet-level Committee on Economic Security. This committee drafted the original Social Security Act, in which Cohen, only twenty-one years old, played a significant role. In 1935 he was a member of the Committee on Public Administration of the Social Science Research Council and eventually became director of the Bureau of Research and Statistics in charge of program development and legislative-coordination work with Congress. In 1960, President-elect John F. Kennedy named Cohen to head up a Task Force on Health and Social Security, which would make recommendations for improving national programs in these areas. Shortly after taking office, President Kennedy appointed Cohen assistant secretary (for legislation) of Health, Education and Welfare; and, in 1968, President Johnson elevated him to director of the department. In these positions, he played a critical role in the development of key health-related legislation, including Medicare and Medicaid. After leaving government service after Nixon's election to the presidency, Cohen continued to be active in trying to influence and support Social Security, eventually founding the Save Our Security coalition.

Ronald Dellums (November 24, 1935–)

Ronald Dellums served as a congressman from California from 1970 to 1998. Although his service in Congress had a strong focus on military and foreign issues, he also introduced in 1977 the National Health Service Act, a proposal that for two decades represented the most comprehensive and progressive healthcare proposal before the Congress. It was the first legislation introduced to Congress that called for the creation of a national health service. This proposal has helped to guide the debate on major healthcare reform over the past few decades.

Marian Wright Edelman (June 6, 1939–)

Marian Wright Edelman is the founder and president of the Children's Defense Fund (CDF), a strong advocacy group for the rights and welfare of children and families. As the issues of poverty, education, and health (including access to healthcare) of America's children are strongly interrelated, Edelman and her advocacy group have been leading efforts to increase the government's efforts to support the welfare of this country's children. Her agency was a major public advocate for the passage of the CHIP (Children's Health Insurance Program) legislation, which many have viewed as the largest expansion of publicly funded healthcare since the passage of Medicare and Medicaid in 1965. This legislation has the potential of greatly reducing the number of uninsured children in the United States, although issues of adequate state funding for the required state matching and enrollment of children may partially limit the success of this effort. Another effort by the CDF has been to modify and increase the comprehensiveness of public-welfare legislation. With major modifications, this effort recently culminated in the passage of the comprehensive child welfare legislation known as the Leave No Child Behind program.

Alain C. Enthoven (September 10, 1930–)

Alain C. Enthoven is considered the creator of the concept of "managed competition," which has developed into the managed care approach of healthcare that has come to dominate healthcare in the 1990s and beyond. Enthoven started his public service as one of Robert McNamara's chief "Whiz Kids" in the 1960s, in the Defense Department. From 1973 on, he has held the Marriner S. Eccles Professorship of Public and Private Management at Stanford University. In 1977, he presented to the Carter administration his "Consumer Choice Health Plan," which he built on the concepts of prepaid group practice plans developed in the 1930s and 1940s and on the health maintenance organization (HMO) strategy pushed in the early 1970s (Enthoven 1977). The plan was based on what he called "regulated competition." He then added to the concept "design proposals to deal with such issues as financing, biased selection, market segmentation, information costs, and equity" (Enthoven 1993). The key to his vision of managed care is competition, with consumers having a choice among competing plans.

References and Further Reading

Enthoven, Alain C. 1977. Consumer Choice Health Plan: A National Health Insurance Proposal. Memorandum to Health, Education, and Welfare Secretary Joseph Califano. September 22.

———. 1993. The History and Principle of Managed Competition. *Health Affairs* Supplement. (March) pp. 22–48.

White, Jane H. 1993. Cutting through the Confusion of Managed Competition. *Health Progress* (March). http://www.chausa.org/PUBS/PUBSART. ASP?ISSUE=HP9303&ARTICLE=H (Accessed on 1 January 2004).

William H. Frist, M.D. (February 22, 1952–)

William H. Frist, M.D., was elected the U.S. Senate majority leader in January of 2003 at the start of the 108th Congress, thus replacing Trent Lott. Frist was the first practicing physician elected to the Senate since 1928. After receiving his A.B. in health policy from the Woodrow Wilson School of Public and International Affairs at Princeton University, Frist obtained his M.D. at Harvard Medical School. Before entering politics (that is, from 1986 to 1993), he headed the Vanderbilt University Medical Center Multi-Organ Transplant Center, where he also performed heart and lung transplants. In 1994, he was elected to the Senate, representing Tennessee. One of his expectations as he became involved in public service was that he would become a key player in healthcare reform legislation, although there was not much focus on healthcare reform in his first eight years in the Senate. He moved up rapidly in the Senate leadership, culminating in his position as Senate majority leader in 2003. Given his background of expertise in health as well as his new Senate leadership position, he is expected to play an important role in helping to formulate Republican suggestions for healthcare reform during George W. Bush's presidency. For the 2003 year in the Senate, these changes will likely include some examination of Medicare and some suggestions on prescription-drug coverage for the elderly.

Newt Gingrich (January 17, 1943–)

Newt Gingrich served as the Speaker of the U.S. House of Representatives from 1995 to 1999 after having led the Republicans in their effort to regain control of the House. He used the fight against the Clinton health reform initiative as a stepping stone to lead the Republicans to that victory as he developed his Contract with America in response to the "big government" approach of the Clinton healthcare proposal. He took responsibility for the Republican election setbacks in 1998 and resigned from the House and from his role as Speaker of the House in early 1999. Since then, he has been working as chief executive officer of The Gingrich Group, a communications and management-consulting firm, and has remained a strong and vocal proponent on national policy issues, including healthcare.

Lister Hill (December 29, 1894– December 21, 1984)

A congressman and senator from Alabama from 1922 to 1968, Lister Hill guided healthcare and medical-research legislation and funding from after World War II to the early 1960s. In 1946, he sponsored the Hill-Burton Act, which introduced the concept of communities obtaining matching federal funds to meet health-care needs. Under this program 9,200 new hospitals, nursing homes, clinics, and public health facilities were constructed throughout the country. The communities were required to provide free indigent care as part of receiving these construction funds. Although a key program that guided the development of healthcare in this country for fifteen years, the Hill-Burton legislation was actually passed in order to head off President Truman's efforts to pass a national healthcare system. In the 1950s, Hill dominated the federal government's development of the National Institutes of Health (NIH) into the world's premier medical-research center. He accomplished this through his dual roles as chair of the Senate Health, Education and Welfare Committee; its Health Subcommittee; and the Health, Education and Welfare Subcommittee of the Senate Appropriations Committee. Thus he was able to guide both the enabling legislations and the appropriations legislation that built the NIH into the world-premier's research center and enabler. During Eisenhower's terms in office, Hill routinely doubled the president's funding recommendation for the NIH's budget.

Lyndon Baines Johnson (August 27, 1908– January 22, 1973)

The thirty-sixth president of the United States was able to facilitate the enactment of major accomplishments in civil rights and in social programs as part of his Great Society programs. Beyond the health area, many major aspects of social legislation dealing with education, welfare, and voting reform were passed. Within health, the Johnson administration was responsible for the enactment of the two major U.S. government programs that still form the fundamental basis for the U.S. government's role in the direct provision of healthcare to Americans. Passage of Medicare legislation provided health insurance all across the United States for the retired segment of the population. The coverage was comparable to that offered by many businesses at the time and was available to all Social Security recipients, independent of the amount of income and wealth they possessed. The Medicaid program provided healthcare coverage to recipients of major welfare programs through a joint federal-state program, and thus it was a benefit linked to a means-tested welfare system. This was part of an expansion of welfare-type benefits that were known as the Great Society initiative.

Edward M. Kennedy (February 22, 1932–)

Edward Kennedy is the youngest brother of John F. Kennedy (thirty-fifth president of the United States) and Robert F. Kennedy (attorney general in JFK's cabinet and presidential contender when he was assassinated in 1968). Edward Kennedy was elected to the U.S. Senate from Massachusetts in 1962 when JFK resigned to run for the presidency. In 2003, he is serving in his seventh term and is the third-most-senior senator in the Senate. Throughout his time in the Senate, he has been a leading Democrat on health-related issues. In the early 1970s, Kennedy introduced legislation for the establishment of a national healthcare system. The legislation was close to proposals President Nixon was developing when his efforts were ended by the Watergate crisis. In recent years, Kennedy was critical in the passage of the Health Insurance Portability and Accountability Act of 1996, which makes it easier for those who change their jobs or lose their jobs to keep their health insurance, and the Children's Health Insurance Program of 1997 (CHIP), which makes health insurance far more widely available to children through age eighteen in all fifty states. He is currently a leader in the Senate in the effort to enact the patients' bill of rights, which is designed to end the abuses of health maintenance organizations (HMOs) and managed care health plans and to provide greater protection for patients and physicians in dealing with insurance companies. He also became a pivotal person in opposition to the Medicare prescription reform bill, which was debated in Congress in November 2003. Although Kennedy had initially positioned himself as being in favor of a bill to provide some type of prescription coverage to the elderly through Medicare, by the time the Bush administration proposal reached Congress, it included a provision to test, in certain large urban areas, Medicare versus some private companies as a way to deliver benefits, and Kennedy led the unsuccessful opposition to the legislation. His opposition was based on the bill only providing limited coverage initially through a card rather than a real prescription benefit; the high costs with extra funds to doctors and hospitals; the lack of cost-control provisions for drugs; and the notion of the testing of Medicare, which could be a first step to the dissolution of the program.

C. Everett Koop (October 14, 1916–)

C. Everett Koop, one of the most influential and controversial surgeon generals, was appointed deputy assistant secretary for Health for the U.S. Public Health Service (PHS) in February 1981 and was sworn in as surgeon general on November 17, 1981. Additionally, he was appointed director of the Office of International Health in May 1982. He served in these positions until his resignation in 1989. After graduating from Cornell Medical School in 1941, Koop spent most of his career before joining the PHS at the University of Pennsylvania School of Medicine. He started there as an intern, then stayed as a graduate student, and then as a faculty member. After promotions up the academic ladder, he was named professor of Pediatric Surgery at the University of Pennsylvania School of Medicine in 1959 and professor of pediatrics in 1971. During this time he also practiced, quickly becoming an internationally respected pediatric surgeon and becoming surgeon-in-chief of the Children's Hospital of Philadelphia in 1948 and serving in that capacity until he left the academic world in 1981. As surgeon general, Dr. Koop was outspoken on health matters such as smoking and health, diet and nutrition, environmental health hazards, and the importance of immunization and disease prevention. He was also the government's leading spokesman about the then-emerging AIDS epidemic. Even though he was known before his government service as a conservative, he strongly advocated, from a public health viewpoint, the importance of sex education in schools.

Philip R. Lee (April 17, 1924–)

Philip R. Lee is senior advisor to the School of Medicine regarding the development of the social, behavioral, and policy sciences at the University of California, San Francisco (UCSF). From July 1993 through January 1997, he served as assistant secretary for health in the U.S. Department of Health and Human Services (DHHS), a post he also held under President Lyndon B. Johnson. In both of these administrations, he was a key advisor for health policy. Before going to Washington, D.C., in 1993, Dr. Lee served as director of the Institute for Health Policy Studies, which he founded at UCSF in 1972 with Lewis H. Butler, L.L.B., and from 1969 to 1972 he was chancellor of UCSF. Dr. Lee has frequently been an advisor to federal, state, and local health policy makers, and has served on numerous advisory boards and in planning groups. Dr. Lee's research and teaching endeavors in the field of health policy have focused on physician payment, prescription drugs, reproductive-health policy, and AIDS-related issues. Currently, he also is doing research on population health, public health, and medical care, particularly the role of multispecialty group practice.

Ira Magaziner (November 8, 1947–)

Ira Magaziner was a key policy advisor and friend to President Clinton. Their association went back twenty-five years to their years together as Rhodes scholars at Oxford University. Along with Hillary Clinton, Magaziner cochaired President Clinton's failed healthcare reform initiative in 1993 and 1994. He subsequently became a key advisor to Clinton on Internet and technology policy. Prior to his White House appointment, Mr. Magaziner earned respect as one of America's most successful corporate strategists, building two successful consulting firms with a focus on corporate strategy and directing policy analysis for major corporations.

Richard Nixon (January 9, 1913–
April 22, 1994)

The thirty-seventh president of the United States is most remembered for his China initiative and his fall from power because of the Watergate scandal. Less well known is the fact that the top priority of his second administration was to be the passage and implementation of a single-payer, national healthcare system. In his first administration in the early 1970s, one of the major overall economic problems was high inflation. To deal with this problem, wage and price controls were instituted, including controls in the healthcare sector. The period of price controls was one of the few periods since 1965 when the growth in costs of healthcare did not exceed the overall rate of inflation. These trends helped to sensitize the major advisors to Nixon and Nixon himself to the importance of instituting some changes in the healthcare system. In 1973, Congress passed Nixon's Health Maintenance Organization (HMO) Act that was focused on increasing the numbers of prepaid group practice plans, which then became renamed as HMOs. After the 1974 election, preliminary discussions with the

Democrats in Congress led to some agreement about the useful-ness of considering major reform along the lines of a single-payer, national healthcare system. Many health policy analysts believe that the positions of the two major political parties, the Demo-crats and the Republicans, were as close to agreement on major reform as they had ever been. However, this growing consensus for reform and change in the healthcare system was shattered by the political crisis of Watergate, which led to impeachment hear-ings. This made health reform another victim of the Watergate break-in.

Ron Pollack (February 21, 1944–)

Ron Pollack is an attorney and activist on public-policy issues. He has been the director of Families USA, an advocacy group representing families. Although families are an important focus of this advocacy group, it has also had a focus on health issues since its inception as the Villers Foundation in 1982. During 1997 and 1998, Pollack was appointed to serve on the Presidential Ad-visory Commission on Consumer Protection and Quality in the Health Care Industry. He was the sole consumer-organization representative on that body. He worked on the preparation of the patients' bill of rights, legislation to help improve the ability of patients to have options and to be able to register formal com-plaints against healthcare insurance companies, healthcare man-agement companies, and other healthcare providers. This legis-lation has been passed in many states and is pending in the U.S. Congress. His organization was one of the groups that pushed for the passage of the Children's Health Insurance Program (CHIP) as a step forward in health insurance coverage for fami-lies through the provision of health insurance coverage to chil-dren of the near poor and working poor. He was also the founder and chair of the Health Assistance Partnership, an entity that works with healthcare ombudsman programs across the country to help consumers navigate the increasingly complex U.S. healthcare system.

Ronald Reagan (February 6, 1911–)

Ronald Reagan was the fortieth president of the United States, serving from 1981 to 1989. The Reagan presidency began the shift from the activist government that had dominated federal policy from Franklin D. Roosevelt until Reagan's presidency. The Reagan Revolution was focused on reducing the government's impact on individuals and reducing their dependence on the government. As an actor from the late 1930s until the early 1960s, Reagan became politically active as a member of the Screen Actors Guild, eventually becoming its president. In this role he shifted his political views from liberal to conservative. In 1966 he was elected to the first of his two terms as governor of California. While conservative and in favor of less federal regulation for health issues in general, a major regulatory-oriented reform, diagnosis-related groups (DRGs), was enacted during Reagan's presidency as a cost-containment measure.

Franklin D. Roosevelt (January 30, 1882– April 12, 1945)

Franklin D. Roosevelt was the thirty-second president of the United States, serving from 1933 until his death in 1945. He is the only president to serve for more than two terms. Roosevelt became president in the depths of the Great Depression. To deal with the unprecedented economic conditions, including massive unemployment, Roosevelt introduced the New Deal, a series of government programs intended to stimulate the economy, create jobs, and help provide relief for various groups of the poor, including unemployed young men, families with unemployed breadwinners, and portions of the elderly. Among the programs introduced, Social Security, which provides basic levels of income support to the elderly, has had the most lasting effect. Although in some of the early discussions, Social Security was going to include a health program (with some similarities to what was eventually passed as the Medicare program in 1965 under President Johnson), as introduced to the Congress, the Social Security legislation did not include a health component. This was left out due to concerns that a health portion would lead to organized opposition to the Social Security legislation from groups such as the American Medical Association (AMA). Although his programs had some limited success economically, the U.S. economy did not totally recover until the outbreak of World War II in 1939. Although Roosevelt did not introduce any programs relating to healthcare due to his concerns about alienating the AMA (which opposed such programs), he greatly expanded the role of the federal government in social-welfare issues, setting the stage for the major expansions of the government role into health with the passage of Medicare and Medicaid in 1965.

Theodore Roosevelt (October 27, 1858– January 16, 1919)

Theodore Roosevelt was the twenty-sixth president of the United States, serving from 1901 to 1909. In 1912, he was the candidate for president on the Progressive Party ticket. He ran on a platform of social reform. His Progressive Party (a creation of Roosevelt's that was more popularly known as the Bull Moose Party) included a health insurance plank in its campaign platform. This was the first inclusion of a health insurance plank in any national platform with a major candidate, although the Socialist Party had endorsed a compulsory system as early as 1904. Many of his ideas about health insurance reform came from the American Association of Labor Legislation (AALL), founded in 1906. This group spearheaded drives for workers' compensation (ultimately successful) and for a government-sponsored health insurance system for the general population (unsuccessful, as was Roosevelt's candidacy in 1912).

Tommy G. Thompson (November 19, 1941–)

Tommy G. Thompson is the current (2003) secretary of the U.S. Department of Health and Human Services (DHHS). As such, he is the leading spokesperson for a variety of health- and welfare-related issues in President George W. Bush's administration. Thompson has spent most of his career in public service in Wisconsin, serving as its governor from 1987 to 2001. During that time, he was part of major welfare reforms within the state of Wisconsin that included a push toward requiring welfare recipients to work. Some of these ideas were part of the change in welfare policy in the United States in 1996 that led to the passage of TANF (Temporary Assistance to Needy Families) to replace programs such as AFDC (Aid to Families with Dependent Children). In 1996, while governor of Wisconsin, Thompson pushed for the enactment of Wisconsin Works, or "W-2," the state's landmark welfare-to-work legislation, which served as a national model for welfare reform. The program required participants to work, while at the same time providing the services and support to make the transition to work feasible and permanent. W-2 provided a safety net through child care, healthcare, transportation, and training assistance. Wisconsin's monthly welfare caseload declined by more than 90 percent, while the economic status of those taking part in W-2 improved. The average family on AFDC had been living at 30 percent below the federal poverty line. However, at the average wage of people leaving W-2, families were 30 percent above the poverty line. After this program was under way, Thompson pushed the state to provide health insurance to many low-income children and families. As of November 2000, the BadgerCare program—Wisconsin's Medicaid/State Children's Health Insurance Program for uninsured families—had enrolled more than 77,000 individuals. In addition, Wisconsin's Pathways to Independence was the nation's first program to allow the disabled to enter the workforce without the fear of losing health benefits. The program provides ready access to a coordinated system of services and benefits counseling. As governor, Thompson also created Family-Care, designed to help elderly and disabled citizens, allowing them to receive care in their homes for as long as possible. Thompson's participation in leading reform in an innovative state in areas of welfare and health reform provides important experience and expertise within the Bush administration.

Harris Wofford (April 9, 1926–)

Harris Wofford was elected to the U.S. Senate from Pennsylvania in a special election in November 1991. In his campaign, he strongly called for reform of the U.S. healthcare system, and his victory was widely seen as an indication of strong support for such reform among the American electorate. His election and its interpretation as a call for healthcare reform were a major impetus for such reform, culminating in President Clinton's failed attempt, partially led by his wife, Hillary (currently the senator from New York), to craft a national health plan in 1993 and 1994. Wofford has a long history of public service, including playing a key role in the founding of the Peace Corps in 1961. Wofford lost his reelection effort for a full term in 1994, but was then appointed by President Clinton as the CEO of the Corporation for National and Community Service, serving in that role from 1995 to 2001.

5

Facts and Documents

Much of the data available in the healthcare area is government data, much of which is collected at the federal level. Although federal agencies have been involved in collection of health-related data for decades, much of this data is more easily available now than ever before. Whereas in the past, government-collected data were available in compiled form in certain libraries that were designated as government repository libraries, most of the more common health-related data that a person might want to consult today is available through a variety of different government-maintained Web sites. In addition to the government Web sites with their focus on data, there are numerous health policy and organizational Web sites that also present data but with more of a policy emphasis. Many of these sites are presented in this chapter and Chapter 6.

Although almost all federal agencies have their own Web sites that display various types of government data, there is now also a specialized Web site, http://www.fedstats.gov, that provides easy access to government information sorted by topics, one of which is health, and by agencies that produce health-related statistics. In the first part of this chapter, descriptions are provided of some of the major data sets and types of data available at the national level, including some explanations of which agencies are responsible for which data sets. For people interested in obtaining data on specific states, some of this is also available through the federal government Web sites. In addition, in some states, state agencies may also have more state or local data available, but this chapter does not attempt to summarize or review the information available through states or local governments. A good overview of health statistics and the problems in finding and using them is presented in the University of Chicago's John Carter Library's Health Statistics Research Guides, located at http://www.lib.uchicago.edu/e/su/med/healthstat.

Federal Agencies and Health-Related Data Collections

Although there are many different federal agencies that may have some information related to health, there are four that contain the most information relevant to healthcare and healthcare reform, and these agencies will be the ones discussed in this chapter. They are the Agency for Health Care Policy and Research (AHCPR), the Centers for Medicare and Medicaid Services (CMS), the Agency for Healthcare Research and Quality (AHRQ), and the National Center for Health Statistics (NCHS) at the Centers for Disease Control and Prevention (CDC).

Of the four major federal agencies that collect health-related data, the most important, with the most data, is the NCHS (http://www.cdc.gov/nchs/), which is part of the CDC. This agency is responsible for the collection, analysis, and dissemination of statistics on the nature and extent of the health, illness, and disability of the U.S. population. This includes gathering information on the impact of illness and disability on the economy; the effects of environmental, social, and other health hazards; the use of healthcare services; health resources; family formation, growth, and dissolution; and vital events (i.e., births and deaths as well as marriages and divorces).

The CDC (http://www.cdc.gov/) provides data on morbidity, infectious and chronic diseases, occupational diseases and injuries, vaccine efficacy, and safety studies. Examples of the more specific things on which data are gathered by this agency include information on the common cold, influenza, asthma, diabetes, disabilities/impairments, health insurance coverage, heart disease, home health/hospice care, hospital utilization, hypertension, child and infant health, mammography/breast cancer, and men's health. In certain of their reports, the NCHS aggregates these data to provide information about the key national indicators of well-being, the leading causes of death, and typical life-expectancy figures for various population groups, all the types of data that are important in determining how well a country's healthcare system is functioning and whether there are important groups within the country, based on geographical criteria or race and ethnicity, that are not having as positive an experience in their overall health and their healthcare.

The AHRQ (formerly AHCPR—Agency for Health Care Policy and Research) (http://www.ahcpr.gov/) produces and disseminates scientific and policy-relevant information about the cost, quality, access, and medical effectiveness of healthcare. Although some data are provided back to 1992, most of the data are presented back to 1996. This agency does much of its work through several special surveys that it conducts. The AHRQ is responsible for the Medical Expenditure Panel Survey (MEPS), a detailed survey that is conducted once every ten years to produce national estimates for a variety of measures related to health status, health insurance coverage, healthcare use and expenditures, and sources of payment for health services. The agency's other major data collection effort is the Healthcare Cost and Utilization Project (HCUP), which collects information using an inpatient sample about hospitalization trends. Through this agency, one can get some instant access to hospital statistics. Special reports are produced, such as a recent *Fact Book No. 3: Care of Women in U.S. Hospitals* (2000). The agency also provides information on quality indications, including information on prevention quality indicators, inpatient quality indicators, and data at a state level for the states that participate in HCUP. There is also information available on state ambulatory-surgery statistics. Another special effort is the Kids' Inpatient Database (KID).

The CMS (http://cms.hhs.gov/) collects administrative data associated with its oversight of the Medicare and Medicaid programs, and also studies the quality of care delivered by those programs. The Health Care Indicators program contains data and analysis of recent trends in healthcare spending, employment, and prices. The National Health Statistics Group tracks trends in healthcare-related industries and presents this information quarterly. These data are valuable for understanding the relationship between the healthcare sector and the overall economy. In addition, they allow the National Health Statistics Group to anticipate the direction and magnitude of healthcare cost changes prior to the availability of more comprehensive data. For the Medicare program, detailed data on many aspects of Medicare enrollment are available, including Medicare National Enrollment Trends for 1966–2001; Medicare State Enrollment: 2001, 2000, and 1999; state enrollment trends for certain years; and some information by county. Data about the Medicaid program and the Children's Health Insurance Program (CHIP) program are also available, but not always as easily or in as much detail as the Medicare data.

The HRSA (http://www.hrsa.gov/) collects data about general health services, the health professions workforce, and resource issues relating to access, equity, quality, and cost of care, and also maintains the Scientific Registry for organ transplants. One of its major data efforts is the *United States Health Workforce Personnel Factbook.* This fact book provides a compilation of data from more than a dozen professional associations and government agencies. From this fact book, a person can learn a great deal about the healthcare workforce. The report covers the current and historical supply of physicians, dentists, nurses, pharmacists, optometrists, podiatrists, and allied health professionals. The fact book also looks toward the future, detailing the number of schools and first-year enrollment patterns for most healthcare disciplines. Trends in practice are depicted in tables that track the number of hospitals, hospital-based personnel, and national healthcare spending over time.

Some other federal agencies that make health-related data available are the following:

- The Indian Health Service (IHS) (http://www.ihs. gov/) has some data, but it is more specialized. The IHS, for example, collects social and economic statistics on all American Indians and Alaska Natives, as well as patient care and morbidity information for those who use IHS services.
- The NIH (National Institutes of Health) (http://www. nih.gov/) supports the design and implementation of epidemiological studies, clinical trials, biomedical research, and laboratory investigations conducted by the various institutes.
- The Office of Environment, Safety, and Health (ESH) (http://tis.eh.doe.gov/portal/home.htm) in the Department of Energy conducts epidemiological studies of the health effects of exposure to radiation and other hazardous substances.
- The Substance Abuse and Mental Health Services Administration (SAMHSA) (http://www.samhsa. gov/) provides information on health problems related

to the use and abuse of drugs and alcohol, substance-abuse treatment, and the mental health condition of the population, and administers and evaluates federal block grants to the states.

These agencies may obtain some federal data, but are not the major sources in the way that the first four agencies are.

Historical Health Data and Government Publications

The best sources for historical data are two government publications—*The Statistical Abstract of the United States,* published annually by the U.S. Census Bureau, and *Health, United States,* published annually by the NCHS.

The Statistical Abstract of the United States (available at http://www.census.gov/prod/www/statistical-abstract-us.html) is the national data book for the United States and contains a collection of statistics on social and economic conditions in the United States. One of its major sections is Section 3, Health and Nutrition. This section presents tables with data by year, with some tables going back as far as 1960 and with many going back as far as 1980. The site provides online access to the abstracts back to 1995.

Health, United States (available at http://www.cdc.gov/nchs/hus.htm) is an annual report on national trends in health statistics. Published annually it provides data in tables on eleven topics relating to healthcare in the United States. The topics in the 2001 edition are:

- population,
- fertility and natality,
- mortality,
- determinants and measures of health,
- ambulatory care,
- inpatient care,
- personnel,
- facilities,
- national health expenditures,
- healthcare coverage and major federal programs, and
- state health expenditures and health insurance.

Many of the tables go back twenty years or more. The annual editions on the Web site are available back to 1975. The next part of this chapter presents nine tables from these two publication with a brief explanation of how to interpret the data presented.

Use of Various Federal and Other Data

Federal data and data from other sources can be presented in a variety of formats. The most common way for data to be displayed is in tables. Sometimes data are displayed in more visually oriented forms. Bar graphs and pie charts are two common visually oriented ways to display data. A good example of pie charts that clearly and easily present data are the two charts displayed in Figure 5.1. These charts, as their titles indicate, display how the nation's dollar was used for healthcare in 2001. The first pie chart shows where the money within the healthcare system came from that year. The second pie chart displays how the nation's healthcare dollar was spent in 2001 and is labeled "Where It Went."

This chapter also includes nine different examples of data tables from federal data sources. These tables are but a sampling of the wealth of data presented in two key federal documents described earlier in this chapter—*The Statistical Abstract of the United States* and *Health, United States*. The tables presented below are from the 2002 edition of *The Statistical Abstract* and the 2003 edition of the *Health, United States* publications. New editions are published on the Web every year, so the Web site should make the most current data available easily accessible.

Table 5.1 presents extensive data on national health expenditures from 1960 to 2000 with projections through 2011. The title presents the subject of the table—a summary of health expenditures in the United States over time. Below the title is an explanation of the scale of the table (each number represents billions of dollars). As with complex tables, this table is made up of several tables put together for comparative purposes. The first and second sections (Private Expenditures and Public Expenditures) give the breakdown of expenditures by source of payment, adding together to make up most of the Total Expenditures column. The third section gives the broad breakdown of most of these expenditures by where they went. Several observations can

FIGURE 5.1
The Nation's Health Dollar: 2001

Where It Came From

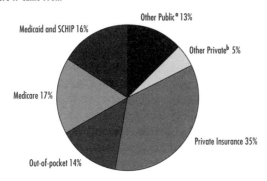

Where It Went

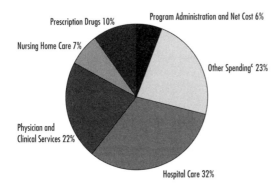

a. "Other Public" includes programs such as workers' compensation, public health activity, Department of Defense, Department of Veterans Affairs, Indian Health Service, and state and local hospital subsidies and school health.
b. "Other Private" includes industrial in-plant, privately funded construction, and non-patient revenues, including philanthropy.
c. "Other Spending" includes dental services, other professional services, home health care, durable medical products, over-the-counter medicines and sundries, public health activities, research, and construction.
Source: Centers for Medicare and Medicaid Services, Office of the Actuary, National Health Statistics Group.

be made from this table. One is the absolute increase in expenditures with an almost fiftyfold increase in the forty years from 1960 to 2000. The growing importance of private insurance is indicated by its rapid growth relative to out-of-pocket expenditures. Also of interest in the Health Services and Supplies part of

TABLE 5.1
National Health Expenditures—Summary, 1960 to 2000, and Projections, 2001 to 2011
(In billions of dollars [27 represents $27,000,000,000]. Includes Puerto Rico and outlying areas.)

Year	Total Expenditures[a]	Private Expenditures			Public Expenditures			Health Services and Supplies				
		Total[b]	Out-of-Pocket	Insurance	Total	Federal	State and Local	Total[c]	Hospital Care	Physician and Clinical Services	Prescription Drugs	Nursing Home Care
1960	27	20	13	6	7	3	4	25	9	5	3	1
1961	29	21	13	7	7	3	4	27	10	6	3	1
1962	31	23	14	7	8	4	4	29	11	6	3	1
1963	34	25	15	8	9	4	5	31	12	7	3	1
1964	38	28	17	9	9	4	5	34	13	8	3	1
1965	41	31	18	10	10	5	6	37	14	8	4	2
1966	45	32	19	10	14	7	6	41	16	9	4	2
1967	51	32	19	11	19	12	7	47	18	10	4	2
1968	58	36	21	12	22	14	8	53	21	11	5	3
1969	65	40	23	13	24	16	9	59	24	12	5	4
1970	73	45	25	16	28	18	10	67	28	14	6	4
1971	81	50	26	18	31	20	11	75	31	16	6	5
1972	91	56	29	21	35	23	12	84	34	17	6	6
1973	101	61	32	23	39	25	14	93	39	19	7	6
1974	114	67	35	26	46	30	16	106	45	22	7	7
1975	130	75	37	30	55	36	19	121	52	25	8	9
1976	149	87	41	37	62	43	20	139	60	28	9	10

(continues)

TABLE 5.1

National Health Expenditures (continued)

Year	Private Expenditures				Public Expenditures			Health Services and Supplies				
	Total Expenditures[a]	Total[b]	Out-of-Pocket	Insurance	Total	Federal	State and Local	Total[c]	Hospital Care	Physician and Clinical Services	Prescription Drugs	Nursing Home Care
1977	169	99	45	45	70	47	23	160	68	33	9	12
1978	189	110	48	52	80	54	26	179	76	35	10	13
1979	214	124	53	60	90	61	29	203	87	41	11	15
1980	246	141	58	68	105	71	34	234	102	47	12	18
1981	285	164	66	81	121	83	39	271	119	55	13	20
1982	321	187	72	94	134	92	42	305	135	61	15	23
1983	354	206	79	104	148	102	46	336	146	68	17	26
1984	390	229	86	118	161	113	48	372	156	77	20	28
1985	427	252	96	130	175	122	52	409	167	90	22	31
1986	457	267	103	135	190	132	59	439	178	100	24	34
1987	498	289	109	148	209	143	66	478	192	112	27	36
1988	558	332	119	175	226	154	72	535	209	127	31	41
1989	623	371	126	205	252	172	79	599	229	142	35	46
1990	696	414	137	234	283	193	90	670	254	158	40	53
1991	762	441	142	254	321	222	99	735	280	175	45	58
1992	827	469	146	274	359	251	107	797	302	190	48	62
1993	888	498	147	298	390	274	116	856	320	201	51	66
1994	937	510	144	312	427	299	129	905	332	211	55	68

(continues)

TABLE 5.1
National Health Expenditures *(continued)*

Year	Total Expenditures[a]	Private Expenditures Total[b]	Out-of-Pocket	Insurance	Public Expenditures Total	Federal	State and Local	Health Services and Supplies Total[c]	Hospital Care	Physician and Clinical Services	Prescription Drugs	Nursing Home Care
1995	990	534	147	330	456	322	134	958	344	221	61	75
1996	1,040	558	152	345	482	344	138	1,006	356	229	67	80
1997	1,091	589	162	359	502	359	144	1,054	368	241	76	85
1998	1,150	629	175	383	521	368	153	1,112	379	257	87	89
1999	1,216	667	184	409	549	385	164	1,175	392	270	104	89
2000	1,300	712	195	444	587	412	176	1,256	412	286	122	92
2001 proj.	1,424	776	210	487	648	453	195	1,377	446	311	142	99
2002 proj.	1,546	849	227	537	697	484	213	1,497	476	336	161	104
2003 proj.	1,653	913	243	580	741	511	230	1,601	502	361	182	107
2004 proj.	1,773	980	259	624	794	546	248	1,718	532	388	204	113
2005 proj.	1,902	1,050	276	672	853	585	268	1,843	565	415	228	120
2006 proj.	2,037	1,121	294	720	916	626	290	1,973	599	443	253	126
2007 proj.	2,175	1,192	311	767	983	670	313	2,107	632	469	280	134
2008 proj.	2,320	1,263	330	813	1,057	719	338	2,248	666	498	309	141
2009 proj.	2,476	1,340	351	862	1,136	771	365	2,399	701	528	341	149
2010 proj.	2,639	1,417	372	912	1,222	828	394	2,557	737	559	376	157
2011 proj.	2,816	1,500	396	966	1,316	891	425	2,728	775	593	414	166

[a]Includes medical research and medical facilities construction, not shown separately. [b]Includes other private expenditures, not shown separately. [c]Includes other objects of expenditure, not shown separately.

Source: U.S. Centers for Medicare and Medicaid Services, "Health Accounts," <http://cms.hhs.gov/statistics/nhe/default.asp>.

the table is the fact that the relative proportion of expenditures in the four categories has not changed dramatically over the fifty years covered by the table. The notes at the bottom explain why the totals are slightly off from the sum of the categories totaled. The source of the data is also presented. These are examples of what can be learned in using data to better understand the healthcare system.

Table 5.2 also relates to national health expenditures, focusing on the type of expenditure. This table, as indicated in the title, provides more details from 1990 to 2000, and includes specific figures for 1990 and for each year from 1994 through 2000. This table provides the annual percentage change, the percent of gross domestic product that health expenditures represent for that specific year, and more details on the sources of expenditures, both private and public. As contrasted with the previous table, this table includes more detail on some of the specific sources of public expenditures, with actual figures for programs such as Medicare and Medicaid.

Table 5.3 provides data about national health expenditures also, again mostly covering the year 1990 and years 1994 to 2000, along with a column for 2001 projections. As contrasted with the previous table, this one provides expenditures by object. This means details are provided for such categories as hospital care, physician and clinical services, dental care, home healthcare, and prescription drugs, along with other categories.

Table 5.4 provides information about average annual expenditures per consumer unit, providing figures for 1985, 1990, 1995, and 1997 through 2000. The figures are also provided by certain basic characteristics of the person, such as age, race, origin, size of consumer unit, and income. Depending on the interest of the reader, this table provides a great deal of information about variation in expenditures. Looking at the age figures, for example, the amount column makes the point clearly that average annual expenditures increase as people become older. Following the various columns, the table also illustrates that this trend of increasing expenditures by age is true for health insurance and drugs and medical supplies, but is not as consistent a pattern for medical services. For that category, people fifty-five to sixty-four have higher expenditures than those sixty-five to seventy-four and seventy-five and over.

Table 5.5 moves away from expenditures and presents simple information about the numbers of people enrolled in

TABLE 5.2
National Health Expenditures by Type: 1990 to 2000
(in billions of dollars [696.0 represents $696,000,000,000], except percent. Includes Puerto Rico and outlying areas)

Type of Expenditure	1990	1994	1995	1996	1997	1998	1999	2000
Total	696.0	937.2	990.3	1040.0	1091.2	1149.8	1215.6	1299.5
Annual percent change[a]	11.8	5.5	5.7	5.0	4.9	5.4	5.7	6.9
Percent of gross domestic product	12.0	13.3	13.4	13.3	13.1	13.1	13.1	13.2
Private expenditures	413.5	510.3	534.1	558.2	588.8	628.8	666.5	712.3
Health services and supplies	401.9	496.8	521.6	545.0	573.9	613.3	651.1	695.6
Out-of-pocket payments	137.3	143.9	146.5	152.1	162.3	174.5	184.4	194.5
Insurance premiums[b]	233.5	312.1	330.1	344.8	359.4	383.2	409.4	443.9
Other	31.1	40.7	44.9	48.2	52.1	55.6	57.3	57.2
Medical research	1.0	1.4	1.4	1.6	1.6	2.0	2.2	2.3
Medical facilities construction	10.7	12.1	11.1	11.6	13.3	13.6	13.3	14.3
Public expenditures	282.5	427.0	456.2	481.8	502.4	520.9	549.0	587.2
Percent federal of public	68.2	69.9	70.6	71.4	71.4	70.6	70.1	70.1
Health services and supplies	267.7	408.0	436.1	460.8	480.1	498.2	524.0	559.9
Medicare[c]	110.2	165.8	182.7	197.5	208.2	209.5	212.6	224.4
Public assistance medical payments[d]	78.7	139.2	149.5	157.6	164.8	176.6	191.8	208.5
Temporary disability insurance[e]	0.1	0.1	0.1	0.1	0.1	0.1	0.1	0.1
Workers' compensation (medical)[e]	17.5	22.2	21.9	21.9	20.5	20.8	22.5	23.3
Defense Dept. hospital, medical	10.4	11.8	12.1	12.0	12.1	12.2	12.5	13.0
Maternal, child health programs	1.8	2.2	2.2	2.3	2.3	2.4	2.5	2.6
Public health activities	20.2	30.0	31.4	33.0	35.5	37.9	40.9	44.2
Veterans' hospital, medical care	11.3	15.1	15.4	16.3	16.3	16.9	17.7	18.9
Medical vocational rehabilitation	0.5	0.7	0.7	0.7	0.7	0.8	0.7	0.8
State and local hospitals[f]	13.1	15.3	14.1	13.6	13.4	14.2	14.8	15.6
Other[g]	3.8	5.6	6.0	6.0	6.1	6.9	7.8	8.7
Medical research	11.7	14.8	15.7	16.2	17.1	18.6	20.9	23.0
Medical facilities construction	3.1	4.2	4.4	4.8	5.2	4.1	4.2	4.3

[a]Change from immediate prior year. For explanation of average annual percent change, see Guide to Tabular Presentation.
[b]Covers insurance benefits and amount retained by insurance companies for expenses, additions to reserves, and profits (net cost of insurance).
[c]Represents expenditures for benefits and administrative cost from federal hospital and medical insurance trust funds under old-age, survivors', disability, and health insurance programs; see text, of this section.
[d]Payments made directly to suppliers of medical care (primarily medicaid).
[e]Includes medical benefits paid under public law by private insurance carriers, state governments, and self-insurers.
[f]Expenditures not offset by other revenues.
[g]Covers expenditures for Substance Abuse and Mental Health Services Administration, Indian Health Service, school health, and other programs.
Source: U.S. Centers for Medicare and Medicaid Services, "Health Accounts," <http://cms.hhs.gov/statistics/nhe/default.asp>.

TABLE 5.3
National Health Expenditures by Object, 1990–2000, and Projections, 2001
(in billions of dollars [696.0 represents $696,000,000,000], except percent. Includes Puerto Rico and outlying areas)

Type of Expenditure	1990	1994	1995	1996	1997	1998	1999	2000	2001 proj.
Total	696.0	937.2	990.3	1,040.0	1,091.2	1,149.8	1,215.6	1,299.5	1,423.8
Spent by—									
Consumers	370.8	456.1	476.7	496.8	521.8	557.7	593.8	638.4	697.1
Out-of-pocket	137.3	143.9	146.5	152.1	162.3	174.5	184.4	194.5	210.4
Private insurance	233.5	312.1	330.1	344.8	359.4	383.2	409.4	443.9	486.7
Government	282.5	427.0	456.2	481.8	502.4	520.9	549.0	587.2	648.1
Other[a]	42.8	54.2	57.4	61.4	67.0	71.1	72.7	73.8	78.6
Spent for—									
Health services and supplies	669.6	904.8	957.7	1,005.7	1,053.9	1,111.5	1,175.0	1,255.5	1,377.3
Personal health care expenses	609.4	816.5	865.7	911.9	959.2	1,009.9	1,062.6	1,130.4	1,235.2
Hospital care	253.9	332.4	343.6	355.9	367.5	379.2	392.2	412.1	446.3
Physician and clinical services	157.5	210.5	220.5	229.4	241.0	256.8	270.2	286.4	310.6
Dental services	31.5	41.4	44.5	46.8	50.2	53.2	56.4	60.0	64.4
Other professional services[b]	18.2	25.7	28.5	30.9	33.4	35.5	36.7	39.0	42.7
Home health care	12.6	26.1	30.5	33.6	34.5	33.6	32.3	32.4	35.9
Prescription drugs	40.3	54.6	60.8	67.2	75.7	87.2	103.9	121.8	141.8
Other nondurable medical products	22.5	24.3	25.6	27.1	27.9	28.6	30.4	31.2	32.8
Durable medical equipment[c]	10.6	13.3	14.2	15.3	16.2	16.5	17.6	18.5	19.9
Nursing home care	52.7	68.3	74.6	79.9	85.1	89.1	89.3	92.2	99.2
Other personal health care	9.6	19.9	22.9	25.8	27.8	30.2	33.7	36.7	41.5

(continues)

TABLE 5.3

National Health Expenditures by Object, 1990–2000, and Projections, 2001 *(continued)*

(in billions of dollars [696.0 represents $696,000,000,000], except percent. Includes Puerto Rico and outlying areas)

Type of Expenditure	1990	1994	1995	1996	1997	1998	1999	2000	2001 proj.
Government administration and net cost of private health insurance[d]	40.0	58.3	60.6	60.9	59.2	63.7	71.5	80.9	92.7
Government public health activities	20.2	30.0	31.4	33.0	33.5	37.9	40.9	44.2	49.5
Medical research[e]	12.7	16.3	17.1	17.8	18.7	20.6	23.1	25.3	26.6
Medical facilities construction	13.7	16.2	15.5	16.4	18.5	17.7	17.5	18.6	19.8

[a]Includes nonpatient revenues, privately funded construction, and industrial inplant.

[b]Includes services of registered and practical nurses in private duty, podiatrists, optometrists, physical therapists, clinical psychologists, chiropractors, naturopaths, and Christian Science practitioners.

[c]Includes expenditures for eyeglasses, hearing aids, orthopedic appliances, artificial limbs, crutches, wheelchairs, etc.

[d]Includes administrative expenses of federally financed health programs.

[e]Research and development expenditures of drug companies and other manufacturers and providers of medical equipment and supplies are excluded from research expenditures, but are included in the expenditure class in which the product falls.

Source: U.S. Centers for Medicare and Medicaid Services, "Health Accounts," <http://cms.hhs.gov/statistics/nhe/default.asp>.

TABLE 5.4
Average Annual Expenditures per Consumer Unit for Health Care: 1985 to 2000 (in dollars, except percent)

Item	Health Care, Total					Percent Distribution		
	Amount	Percent of Total Expenditures	Health Insurance	Medical Services	Drugs and Medical Supplies[a]	Health Insurance	Medical Services	Drugs and Medical Supplies[a]
1985	1,108	4.7	375	496	238	33.8	44.8	21.5
1990	1,480	5.2	581	562	337	39.3	38.0	22.8
1995	1,732	5.4	860	512	360	49.7	29.6	20.8
1997	1,841	5.3	881	531	428	47.9	28.8	23.2
1998	1,903	5.4	913	542	448	48.0	28.5	23.5
1999	1,959	5.3	923	558	479	47.1	28.5	24.5
2000	2,066	5.4	983	568	515	47.6	27.5	24.9
Age of reference person:								
Under 25 years old	504	2.2	211	178	115	41.9	35.3	22.8
25 to 34 years old	1,256	3.2	640	367	250	51.0	29.2	19.9
35 to 44 years old	1,774	3.9	850	555	369	47.9	31.3	20.8
45 to 54 years old	2,200	4.8	976	699	525	44.4	31.8	23.9
55 to 64 years old	2,508	6.4	1,132	721	655	45.1	28.7	26.1
65 to 74 years old	3,163	10.3	1,608	686	870	50.8	21.7	27.5
75 years old and older	3,338	15.2	1,631	658	1,049	48.9	19.7	31.4
Race of reference person:								
White and other	2,198	5.6	1,030	620	548	46.9	28.2	24.9
Black	1,107	3.9	639	191	276	57.7	17.3	24.9

(continues)

TABLE 5.4
Average Annual Expenditures per Consumer Unit for Health Care: 1985 to 2000 (in dollars, except percent) (continued)

Item	Health Care, Total		Health Insurance	Medical Services	Drugs and Medical Supplies[a]	Percent Distribution		
	Amount	Percent of Total Expenditures	Health Insurance	Medical Services	Drugs and Medical Supplies[a]	Health Insurance	Medical Services	Drugs and Medical Supplies[a]
Origin of reference person:								
Hispanic	1,243	3.8	600	364	280	48.3	29.3	22.5
Non-Hispanic	2,144	5.6	1,019	587	538	47.2	27.4	25.1
Region of residence:								
Northeast	1,862	4.8	908	504	450	48.8	27.1	24.2
Midwest	2,172	5.5	1,047	575	550	48.2	26.5	25.3
South	2,147	6.2	1,063	533	552	49.5	24.8	25.7
West	2,001	4.8	853	669	479	42.6	33.4	23.9
Size of consumer unit:								
One person	1,488	6.5	657	418	413	44.2	28.1	27.8
Two or more persons	2,307	5.2	1,119	631	557	48.5	27.4	24.1
Two persons	2,596	6.7	1,241	663	692	47.8	25.5	26.7
Three persons	2,080	4.6	1,031	575	474	49.6	27.6	22.8
Four persons	2,143	4.1	1,062	651	429	49.6	30.4	20.0
Five persons or more	2,018	4.1	970	588	460	48.1	29.1	22.8
Income before taxes:								
Complete income reporters[b]	2,120	5.3	985	583	552	46.5	27.5	26.0
Quintiles of income:								
Lowest 20 percent	1,470	8.2	690	339	441	46.9	23.1	30.0

(continues)

TABLE 5.4

Average Annual Expenditures per Consumer Unit for Health Care: 1985 to 2000 (in dollars, except percent) (continued)

Item	Health Care, Total					Percent Distribution		
	Amount	Percent of Total Expenditures	Health Insurance	Medical Services	Drugs and Medical Supplies[a]	Health Insurance	Medical Services	Drugs and Medical Supplies[a]
Second 20 percent	1,968	7.5	945	424	619	47.5	21.3	31.1
Third 20 percent	1,964	5.7	943	524	497	48.0	26.7	25.3
Fourth 20 percent	2,312	4.9	1,090	659	563	47.1	28.5	24.4
Highest 20 percent	2,864	3.8	1,254	968	642	43.8	33.8	22.4
Incomplete reporters of income	1,919	6.0	977	524	419	50.9	27.3	21.8

[a]Includes prescription and nonprescription drugs.
[b]A complete reporter is a consumer unit providing values for at least one of the major sources of income.
Source: Bureau of Labor Statistics, *Consumer Expenditure Survey,* annual.

TABLE 5.5
Medicare Enrollees: 1980 to 2000
(in millions [28.5 represents 28,500,000]. As of July 1. Includes Puerto Rico and
outlying areas and enrollees in foreign countries and unknown place of residence)

Item	1980	1985	1990	1995	1997	1998	1999	2000
Total	28.5	31.1	34.2	37.5	38.4	38.8	39.1	39.6
Aged	25.5	28.2	30.9	33.1	33.6	33.8	33.9	34.2
Disabled	3.0	2.9	3.3	4.4	4.8	5.0	5.2	5.4
Hospital insurance	28.1	30.6	33.7	37.1	38.1	38.4	38.7	39.2
Aged	25.1	27.7	30.5	32.7	33.2	33.4	33.5	33.8
Disabled	3.0	2.9	3.3	4.4	4.8	5.0	5.2	5.4
Supplementary medical insurance	27.4	30.0	32.6	35.7	36.5	36.8	37.0	37.4
Aged	24.7	27.3	29.7	31.7	32.2	32.3	32.4	32.6
Disabled	2.7	2.7	2.9	3.9	4.3	4.5	4.6	4.8

Source: U.S. Centers for Medicare and Medicaid Services, Office of the Actuary, "Medicare Enrollment Trends 1966–1999"; published 16 November 2000; <http://www.hcfa.gov/stats/enrllmd.htm> and unpublished data.

Medicare from 1980 to 2000. Numbers are presented for those who are in both the aged and disabled categories, and figures are also provided for those with hospital insurance coverage and also for those with supplemental medical insurance.

Tables 5.6 through 5.8 provide information about health insurance coverage or the lack of such coverage. Table 5.6 provides figures on health insurance coverage status for 1990 to 2000 by such characteristics as age, sex, race, and household income. Actual numbers are provided along with percentages, and figures are presented for coverage by private or government health insurance. Looking at the income breakdowns, for example, the percentage covered by any insurance increases as income increases. This is because as income increases, the percentage of private health insurance increases from 41 percent for those earning less than $25,000 to 90 percent for those earning $75,000 or more. In contrast, the highest percentage of people with Medicaid coverage are those in the lowest income category.

Table 5.7 also includes information on persons with and without health insurance coverage, but provides information for one year, 2000. Rather than examining these figures by individual characteristics, this table focuses on variation by state and also provides information about all persons not covered and specifically about whether children are covered.

TABLE 5.6
Health Insurance Coverage Status by Selected Characteristics: 1990 to 2000

(Persons as of following year for coverage in the year shown [248.9 represents 248,900,000]. Government health insurance includes Medicare, Medicaid, and military plans.)

Characteristic	Total Persons	Number (mil.) Total[a]	Covered by Private or Government Health Insurance — Private Total	Group Health[b]	Medicare	Medicaid[c]	Not Covered by Health Insurance	Percent Total[a]	Covered by Private or Government Health Insurance — Private	Medicaid[c]	Not Covered by Health Insurance
1990	248.9	214.2	182.1	150.2	32.3	24.3	34.7	86.1	73.2	9.7	13.9
1995[d]	264.3	223.7	185.9	161.5	34.7	31.9	40.6	84.6	70.3	12.1	15.4
1999[d]	274.1	231.5	194.6	172.0	36.1	27.9	42.6	84.5	71.0	10.2	15.5
1999[d, e]	274.1	234.8	197.5	174.1	36.1	28.2	39.3	85.7	72.1	10.3	14.3
2000, total[d, e, f]	276.5	237.9	200.2	177.3	37.0	28.6	38.7	86.0	72.4	10.4	14.0
Age:											
Under 18 years	72.6	64.1	51.2	48.1	0.5	14.7	8.4	88.4	70.6	20.3	11.6
Under 6 years	23.7	21.0	15.9	15.3	0.2	5.7	2.6	88.9	67.1	24.2	11.1
6 to 11 years	24.8	22.0	17.5	16.6	0.1	5.1	2.8	88.5	70.5	20.6	11.5
12 to 17 years	24.1	21.1	17.8	16.2	0.2	3.9	2.9	87.8	74.0	16.2	12.2
18 to 24 years	27.0	19.6	17.5	14.4	0.2	2.3	7.4	72.7	64.8	8.7	27.3
25 to 34 years	37.4	29.5	27.0	25.5	0.4	2.4	7.9	78.8	72.1	6.3	21.2
35 to 44 years	44.8	37.8	35.2	33.3	0.8	2.4	6.9	84.5	78.6	5.4	15.5

(continues)

TABLE 5.6
Health Insurance Coverage Status by Selected Characteristics: 1990 to 2000 *(continued)*
(Persons as of following year for coverage in the year shown [248.9 represents 248,900,000].
Government health insurance includes Medicare, Medicaid, and military plans.)

Characteristic	Total Persons	Number (mil.)							Percent			
		Covered by Private or Government Health Insurance						Not Covered by Health Insurance	Covered by Private or Government Health Insurance			Not Covered by Health Insurance
		Total[a]	Private		Government				Total[a]	Private	Medicaid[c]	
			Total	Group Health[b]	Medicare	Medicaid[c]						
45 to 54 years	38.0	33.5	31.1	29.0	1.3	1.9	4.6	88.0	81.6	4.9	12.0
55 to 64 years	23.8	20.5	18.0	15.9	2.1	1.6	3.2	86.3	75.8	6.8	13.7
65 years and older	33.0	32.7	20.3	11.2	31.7	3.3	0.2	99.3	61.5	10.0	0.7
Sex: Male	135.2	115.1	98.4	88.3	16.2	12.7	20.1	85.1	72.8	9.4	14.9
Female	141.3	122.8	101.8	89.0	20.8	15.9	18.5	86.9	72.1	11.3	13.1
Race: White	226.4	197.2	169.8	149.3	32.0	19.4	29.2	87.1	75.0	8.6	12.9
Black	35.9	29.3	21.2	19.6	3.8	7.3	6.6	81.5	58.9	20.3	18.5
Asian and Pacific Islander	11.3	9.3	7.9	7.1	0.9	1.3	2.0	82.0	69.9	11.3	18.0
Hispanic origin[d]	33.9	23.0	16.3	15.1	2.2	6.3	10.8	68.0	47.9	18.6	32.0
Household income:												
Less than $25,000	61.1	47.2	25.2	16.9	17.6	16.9	13.9	77.3	41.2	27.7	22.7
$25,000–$49,999	75.4	62.6	52.9	45.9	11.1	7.4	12.8	83.0	70.2	9.8	17.0
$50,000–$74,999	59.3	52.8	49.4	45.9	4.2	2.5	6.5	89.0	83.3	4.3	11.0

(continues)

TABLE 5.6

Health Insurance Coverage Status by Selected Characteristics: 1990 to 2000 (continued)

(Persons as of following year for coverage in the year shown [248.9 represents 248,900,000]. Government health insurance includes Medicare, Medicaid, and military plans.)

		Number (mil.)							Percent			
		Covered by Private or Government Health Insurance							Covered by Private or Government Health Insurance			
			Private		Government							
Characteristic	Total Persons	Total^a	Total	Group Health^b	Medicare	Medicaid^c	Not Covered by Health Insurance	Total^a	Private	Medicaid^c	Not Covered by Health Insurance
$75,000 or more	80.8	75.3	72.8	68.6	4.2	1.7	5.5	93.1	90.1	2.2	6.9
Persons below poverty	31.1	21.9	8.6	5.8	4.6	12.3	9.2	70.4	27.8	39.8	29.6

aIncludes other government insurance, not shown separately. Persons with coverage counted only once in total, even though they may have been covered by more than one type of policy.

bRelated to employment of self or other family members.

cBeginning 1997, persons with no coverage other than access to Indian Health Service are no longer considered covered by health insurance; instead they are considered to be uninsured. The effect of this change on the overall estimates of health insurance coverage is negligible; however, the decrease in the number of people covered by Medicaid may be partially due to this change.

dData based on 1990 census adjusted population controls.

eEstimates reflect results of follow-up verification questions.

fIncludes other races not shown separately.

gPersons of Hispanic origin may be of any race.

Source: U.S. Census Bureau; Current Population Reports, P60-215; and unpublished data.

TABLE 5.7
Persons with and without Health Insurance Coverage by State: 2000
(237,857 represents 237,857,000.)

State	Total Persons Covered (1,000)	Total Persons Not Covered Number (1,000)	Total Persons Not Covered Percent of Total	Total Children Not Covered Number (1,000)	Total Children Not Covered Percent of Total
U.S.	237,857	38,683	14.0	8,405	11.6
AL	3,851	600	13.5	98	8.5
AK	522	125	19.3	38	17.7
AZ	4,124	793	16.1	173	12.8
AR	2,261	364	13.9	82	11.6
CA	28,454	6,281	18.1	1,507	15.4
CO	3,665	563	13.3	154	13.7
CT	3,056	263	7.9	22	2.6
DE	705	82	10.4	15	7.2
DC	434	73	14.4	10	9.9
FL	12,537	2,620	17.3	570	16.5
GA	6,638	1,135	14.6	154	8.1
HI	1,039	117	10.1	23	8.3
ID	1,061	196	15.6	51	14.7
IL	10,627	1,659	13.5	371	10.8
IN	5,117	701	12.1	201	13.9
IA	2,615	248	8.7	46	6.2
KS	2,306	301	11.5	75	11.3
KY	3,462	513	12.9	73	7.7
LA	3,423	810	19.1	162	15.7
ME	1,121	145	11.5	22	7.8
MD	4,618	501	9.8	92	7.4
MA	5,661	595	9.5	124	7.8
MI	8,964	982	9.9	179	6.7
MN	4,354	430	9.0	117	9.3
MS	2,425	364	13.1	71	9.2
MO	4,930	586	10.6	124	8.5
MT	714	162	18.5	39	18.7
NE	1,494	164	9.9	40	8.8
NV	1,680	311	15.6	90	14.9
NH	1,155	85	6.8	23	7.0
NJ	7,257	1,049	12.6	203	9.3
NM	1,366	427	23.8	105	20.2
NY	15,608	2,802	15.2	486	10.5
NC	6,541	980	13.0	187	10.1
ND	538	69	11.3	18	11.9

(continues)

TABLE 5.7
Persons with and without Health Insurance Coverage by State: 2000 (continued)
(237,857 represents 237,857,000.)

State	Total Persons Covered (1,000)	Total Persons Not Covered Number (1,000)	Total Persons Not Covered Percent of Total	Total Children Not Covered Number (1,000)	Total Children Not Covered Percent of Total	State	Total Persons Covered (1,000)	Total Persons Not Covered Number (1,000)	Total Persons Not Covered Percent of Total	Total Children Not Covered Number (1,000)	Total Children Not Covered Percent of Total
OH	10,284	1,255	10.9	309	9.5	TX	16,167	4,425	21.5	1,273	21.5
OK	2,651	636	19.3	134	16.8	UT	1,913	296	13.4	75	10.1
OR	2,935	465	13.7	111	12.9	VT	564	67	10.7	15	8.5
PA	11,063	905	7.6	145	4.9	VA	6,091	886	12.7	206	11.7
RI	881	55	5.9	5	2.5	WA	5,075	780	13.3	126	8.1
SC	3,321	448	11.9	68	8.6	WV	1,524	254	14.3	37	9.8
SD	615	82	11.8	20	11.6	WI	5,032	386	7.1	56	3.7
TN	5,003	577	10.3	63	4.7	WY	418	70	14.4	16	12.5

Source: U.S. Census Bureau; Current Population Reports, P60-215; and unpublished data.

The third table on healthcare insurance coverage, Table 5.8, provides information about healthcare coverage for people under sixty-five years of age for the years from 1984 to 2000. Greater details are provided on race and Hispanic origin, and information is provided about all ages and those under eighteen as related to percent of poverty level.

Table 5.9 presents different health-related data. This table provides information on life expectancy at birth, as well as at ages 65 and 75, according to race and sex. Depending upon the age group, different years are covered. The broadest coverage is at birth, with figures provided for 1900, each decade from 1950 through 1990, and 1990 through 2000. The information is presented for all races, for whites, and for blacks. Within each of these groups, the life expectancy figure is provided for both sexes together, and for males and females separately. By comparing sets of figures, for example, it is clear that black female life expectancy is now closer to that of white females (a gap of 5.1 years in 2000) than is true for black males (6.6 years), whereas in 1950 the gap for females was 9.3 years and for males was 7.4 years.

These tables are examples of the vast wealth of data provided by the federal government. These tables were selected both to provide an example of the type of data available and because together they provide a good starting point in the use of data to understand the state of the United States' healthcare system and why there is such interest in its reform. Also, remember that these two publications are updated annually, so go online to retrieve the most up-to-date data available.

Nonprofit Think Tanks' and Policy Coalitions' Data and Documents

The healthcare industry represents more than 15 percent of the U.S. economy and is vital to all citizens. Therefore there are many nonprofit issue-advocacy groups representing the various players such as physicians, consumers, government policy makers, insurance companies, and so forth. The Web sites maintained by these groups contain news, analysis, and data relating to the healthcare system and to health reform, and they are thus another excellent source for summary data and statistics on healthcare and reform. Although these sites represent a specific

TABLE 5.8

No Health Care Coverage among Persons under 65 Years of Age, According to Selected Characteristics: United States, Selected Years 1984–2000

(Data are based on household interviews of a sample of the civilian noninstitutionalized population)

Characteristic	1984	1989	1994[a]	1995	1996	1997[a]	1998	1999	2000
Number in millions:									
Total[b]	29.8	33.4	40.0	37.1	38.6	41.0	30.2	38.5	40.5
Percent of population:									
Total, age adjusted[b, c]	14.3	15.3	17.2	15.9	16.5	17.4	16.5	16.1	16.8
Total, crude[b]	14.5	15.6	17.5	16.1	16.6	17.5	16.6	16.1	16.8
Age:									
Under 18 years	13.9	14.7	15.0	13.4	13.2	14.0	12.7	11.9	12.4
Under 6 years	14.9	15.1	13.4	11.8	11.7	12.5	11.5	11.0	11.7
6–17 years	13.4	14.5	15.8	14.3	13.9	14.7	13.3	12.3	12.8
18–44 years	17.1	18.4	21.7	20.4	21.1	22.4	21.4	21.0	22.0
18–24 years	25.0	27.1	30.8	28.0	29.3	30.1	29.0	27.4	29.7
25–34 years	16.2	18.3	21.9	21.1	22.4	23.8	22.2	22.1	22.7
35–44 years	11.2	12.3	15.9	15.1	15.2	16.7	16.4	16.3	16.8
45–64 years	9.6	10.5	12.0	10.9	12.1	12.4	12.2	12.2	12.7
45–54 years	10.5	11.0	12.5	11.6	12.4	12.8	12.6	12.8	12.8
55–64 years	8.7	10.0	11.2	9.9	11.6	11.8	11.4	11.4	12.5
Sex:[c]									
Male	15.0	16.4	18.5	17.2	17.8	18.5	17.5	17.2	17.8
Female	13.6	14.3	16.1	14.6	15.2	16.2	15.5	15.0	15.8

(continues)

TABLE 5.8

No Health Care Coverage among Persons under 65 Years of Age, According to Selected Characteristics: United States, Selected Years 1984–2000 (continued)

(Data are based on household interviews of a sample of the civilian noninstitutionalized population)

Characteristic	1984	1989	1994[a]	1995	1996	1997[a]	1998	1999	2000
Race:[c, d]									
White only	13.4	14.2	16.6	15.3	15.8	16.3	15.2	14.6	15.2
Black or African American only	20.0	21.4	19.7	18.2	19.6	20.2	20.7	19.5	20.0
American Indian and Alaska Native only	#	#	#	#	#	#	#	38.3	38.2
Asian only	18.0	18.5	20.1	18.2	19.0	19.3	18.1	16.4	17.3
Native Hawaiian and Other Pacific Islander only	---	---	---	---	---	---	---	*	*
2 or more races	---	---	---	---	---	---	---	16.8	18.4
Hispanic origin and race:[c, d]									
Hispanic or Latino	29.1	32.4	31.8	31.5	32.4	34.3	34.0	33.9	35.4
Mexican	33.2	38.8	36.2	36.2	37.5	39.2	40.0	38.0	39.9
Puerto Rican	18.1	23.3	15.7	18.3	15.1	19.4	19.4	19.8	16.4
Cuban	21.6	20.9	27.4	22.1	18.8	20.5	18.4	19.7	25.2
Other Hispanic or Latino	27.5	25.2	30.7	29.7	30.5	32.9	31.1	30.8	32.7
Not Hispanic or Latino	#	#	#	#	#	#	#	13.5	14.1
White only	11.8	11.9	14.4	12.9	13.3	13.7	12.5	12.1	12.5
Black or African American only	19.7	21.3	19.3	18.1	19.5	20.1	20.7	19.4	20.0
Age and percent of poverty level:[e]									
All ages:[c]	34.7	35.8	33.1	31.7	34.5	34.4	34.6	34.4	34.2
Below 100 percent	27.0	31.3	35.0	31.7	33.3	36.1	36.5	35.8	36.5
100–149 percent	17.4	21.8	26.1	24.0	24.3	25.9	26.7	27.7	27.3

(continues)

TABLE 5.8
No Health Care Coverage among Persons under 65 Years of Age, According to Selected Characteristics: United States, Selected Years 1984–2000 (continued)
(Data are based on household interviews of a sample of the civilian noninstitutionalized population)

Characteristic	1984	1989	1994[a]	1995	1996	1997[a]	1998	1999	2000
150–199 percent	5.8	6.8	9.2	8.6	8.6	8.8	8.0	7.7	8.7
200 percent or more	28.9	31.6	22.1	20.0	21.0	22.4	21.5	21.6	20.4
Under 18 years:									
100–149 percent	22.8	26.1	27.7	24.8	25.0	26.1	28.0	24.9	25.6
150–199 percent	12.7	15.8	19.1	18.0	16.0	19.7	17.3	18.8	16.8
200 percent or more	4.2	4.4	7.1	6.4	6.1	6.1	5.0	4.4	5.5
Geographic region:[c]									
Northeast	10.1	10.7	13.6	13.1	13.5	13.4	12.3	12.2	12.1
Midwest	11.1	10.5	12.2	12.1	12.2	13.1	11.9	11.5	12.3
South	17.4	19.4	21.0	19.2	20.0	20.7	20.0	19.8	20.4
West	17.8	18.4	20.4	17.7	18.6	20.4	19.9	18.6	20.2
Location of residence:[c]									
Within MSA[f]	13.3	14.9	16.7	15.2	15.6	16.7	15.8	15.3	16.3
Outside MSA[f]	16.4	16.9	19.0	18.7	19.7	19.9	19.2	18.9	18.8

#Estimates calculated upon request.

*Estimates are considered unreliable. Data not shown to have a relative standard of error of greater than 30 percent.

—Data not available.

[a]The questionnaire changed compared with previous years.

[b]Includes all other races not shown separately and unknown poverty level.

[c]Estimates are age adjusted to the year 2000 standard using three age groups: under 18 years, 18–44 years, and 45–64 years.

[d]Starting with data year 1999, estimates by race and Hispanic origin are tabulated using the 1997 Standards for federal data on race and ethnicity; prior to data year 1999 the 1977 Standards are used

(continues)

TABLE 5.8

No Health Care Coverage among Persons under 65 Years of Age, According to Selected Characteristics: United States, Selected Years 1984–2000 *(continued)*
(Data are based on household interviews of a sample of the civilian noninstitutionalized population)

Estimates for specific race groups are shown when they meet requirements for statistical reliability and confidentiality. Starting with data year 1999, the categories "White only," "Black or African American only," "American Indian and Alaska Native (AI/AN) only," "Asian only," and "Native Hawaiian and Other Pacific Islander only" include persons who reported only one racial group; and the category "2 or more races" includes persons who reported more than one of the five racial groups in the 1997 Standards or one of the five racial groups and "Some other race." Prior to data year 1999, estimates for the race categories shown include persons who reported one race or who reported more than one race and identified one race as best representing their race; and the category "Asian only" includes Native Hawaiian and Other Pacific Islander. Because of the differences between the two Standards, race-specific estimates starting with data year 1999 are not strictly comparable with estimates for earlier years.

To estimate change between 1998 and 1999, race-specific estimates for 1999 based on the 1977 Standards can be used. In comparison with the 1999 estimates based on the 1997 Standards, estimates of the age-adjusted percent with no health coverage based on the 1977 Standards are: 0.1 percentage points higher for the white group; identical for the black group; 0.1 percentage points lower for the Asian and Pacific Islander group; and 1.5 percentage points higher for the AI/AN group.

[a]Prior to 1997 percent of poverty level is based on family income and family size using Bureau of the Census poverty thresholds. Beginning in 1997 percent of poverty level is based on family income, family size, number of children in the family, and, for families with two or fewer adults, the age of the adults in the family. Missing family income data were imputed for 17 percent of the sample under 65 years of age in 1994, 15 percent in 1995, and 16 percent in 1996. Percent of poverty level was unknown for 19 percent of the sample persons under 65 in 1997, 24 percent in 1998, 27 percent in 1999, and 26 percent in 2000.

[b]MSA is metropolitan statistical area.

Notes: Persons not covered by private insurance, Medicaid, Child Health Insurance Program (CHIP), public assistance (through 1996), state-sponsored or other government-sponsored health plans (starting in 1997), Medicare, or military plans are included.

Sources: Centers for Disease Control and Prevention, National Center for Health Statistics, *National Health Interview Survey,* health insurance supplements (1984, 1989, 1994–1996). Starting in 1997 data are from the family core questionnaires.

TABLE 5.9
Life Expectancy at Birth, at 65 Years of Age, and at 75 Years of Age,
According to Race and Sex: United States, Selected Years 1900–2000
(Data are based on death certificates)

Specified Age and Year	All Races			White			Black[a]		
	Both Sexes	Male	Female	Both Sexes	Male	Female	Both Sexes	Male	Female
At birth									
1900[b, c]	47.3	46.3	48.3	47.6	46.6	48.7	33.0	32.5	33.5
1950[c]	68.2	65.6	71.1	69.1	66.5	72.2	60.8	59.1	62.9
1960[c]	69.7	66.6	73.1	70.6	67.4	74.1	63.6	61.1	66.3
1970	70.8	67.1	74.7	71.7	68.0	75.6	64.1	60.0	68.3
1980	73.7	70.0	77.4	74.4	70.7	78.1	68.1	63.8	72.5
1985	74.7	71.1	78.2	75.3	71.8	78.7	69.3	65.0	73.4
1990	75.4	71.8	78.8	76.1	72.7	79.4	69.1	64.5	73.6
1991	75.5	72.0	78.9	76.3	72.9	79.6	69.3	64.6	73.8
1992	75.8	72.3	79.1	76.5	73.2	79.8	69.6	65.0	73.9
1993	75.5	72.2	78.8	76.3	73.1	79.5	69.2	64.6	73.7
1994	75.7	72.4	79.0	76.5	73.3	79.6	69.5	64.9	73.9
1995	75.8	72.5	78.9	76.5	73.4	79.6	69.6	65.2	73.9
1996	76.1	73.1	79.1	76.8	73.9	79.7	70.2	66.1	74.2
1997	76.5	73.6	79.4	77.1	74.3	79.9	71.1	67.2	74.7
1998	76.7	73.8	79.5	77.3	74.5	80.0	71.3	67.6	74.8
1999	76.7	73.9	79.4	77.3	74.6	79.9	71.4	67.8	74.7
2000	76.9	74.1	79.5	77.4	74.8	80.0	71.7	68.2	74.9
At 65 years									
1950[b]	13.9	12.8	15.0	---	12.8	15.1	13.9	12.7	14.9
1960[b]	14.3	12.8	15.8	14.4	12.9	15.9	13.9	12.7	15.1
1970	15.2	13.1	17.0	15.2	13.1	17.1	14.2	12.5	15.7
1980	16.4	14.1	18.3	16.5	14.2	18.4	15.1	13.0	16.8
1985	16.7	14.5	18.5	16.8	14.5	18.7	15.2	13.0	16.9
1990	17.2	15.1	18.9	17.3	15.2	19.1	15.4	13.2	17.2
1991	17.4	15.3	19.1	17.5	15.4	19.2	15.5	13.4	17.2
1992	17.5	15.4	19.2	17.6	15.5	19.3	15.7	13.5	17.4
1993	17.3	15.3	18.9	17.4	15.4	19.0	15.5	13.4	17.1
1994	17.4	15.5	19.0	17.5	15.6	19.1	15.7	13.6	17.2
1995	17.4	15.6	18.9	17.6	15.7	19.1	15.6	13.6	17.1
1996	17.5	15.7	19.0	17.6	15.8	19.1	15.8	13.9	17.2
1997	17.7	15.9	1902	17.8	16.0	19.3	16.1	14.2	17.6
1998	17.8	16.0	19.2	17.8	16.1	19.3	16.1	14.3	17.4
1999	17.7	16.1	19.1	17.8	16.1	19.2	16.0	14.3	17.3
2000	17.9	16.3	19.2	17.9	16.3	19.2	16.2	14.5	17.4
At 75 years									
1980	10.4	8.8	11.5	10.4	8.8	11.5	9.7	8.3	10.7
1985	10.6	9.0	11.7	10.6	9.0	11.7	10.1	8.7	11.1
1990	10.9	9.4	12.0	11.0	9.4	12.0	10.2	8.6	11.2

(continues)

TABLE 5.9
Life Expectancy at Birth, at 65 Years of Age, and at 75 Years of Age,
According to Race and Sex: United States, Selected Years 1900–2000 *(continued)*
(Data are based on death certificates)

Specified Age and Year	All Races			White			Black[a]		
	Both Sexes	Male	Female	Both Sexes	Male	Female	Both Sexes	Male	Female
1991	11.1	9.5	12.1	11.1	9.5	12.1	10.2	8.7	11.2
1992	11.2	9.6	12.2	11.2	9.6	12.2	10.4	8.9	11.4
1993	10.9	9.5	11.9	11.0	9.5	12.0	10.2	8.7	11.1
1994	11.0	9.6	12.0	11.1	9.6	12.0	10.3	8.9	11.2
1995	11.0	9.7	11.9	11.1	9.7	12.0	10.2	8.8	11.1
1996	11.1	9.8	12.0	11.1	9.8	12.0	10.3	9.0	11.2
1997	11.2	9.9	12.1	11.2	9.9	12.1	10.7	9.3	11.5
1998	11.3	10.0	12.2	11.3	10.0	12.2	10.5	9.2	11.3
1999	11.2	10.0	12.1	11.2	10.0	12.1	10.4	9.2	11.1
2000	11.3	10.1	12.1	11.3	10.1	12.1	10.5	9.4	11.2

[a]Data shown for 1900–1960 are for the nonwhite population.
[b]Death registration area only. The death registration area increased from 10 states and the District of Columbia in 1900 to the coterminus United States in 1933.
[c]Includes deaths of persons who were not residents of the 50 states and the District of Columbia.
Notes: Beginning in 1997 life table methodology was revised to construct complete life tables by single years of age that extend to age 100. (Anderson RN. Method for Constructing Complete Annual U.S. Life Tables. National Center for Health Statistics. Vital Health Stat 2(129). 1999.) Previously abridged life tables were constructed for 5-year age groups ending with the age group 85 years and older. Data for additional years are available.
Sources: Centers for Disease Control and Prevention, National Center for Health Statistics, National Vital Statistics System; Grove RD and Hetzel AM, Vital Statistics Rates in the United States, 1940–1960. DHEW Pub. No. (PHS) 1677, Public Health Service, Washington: U.S. Government Printing Office, 1968; life expectancy trend data available at www.cdc.gov/nchs/about/major/dvs/mortdata.htm; Minino AM, Arias E, Kochanek KD, Murphy SL, Smith BL, Deaths: Final data for 2000. National vital statistics reports, vol. 50 no 15. Hyattsville, Maryland: National Center for Health Statistics, 2002.

viewpoint or a specific component of the healthcare system, they can be very useful in understanding different issues relating to healthcare reform as long as the reader remembers the specific viewpoint they represent. The following is information on many of these organizations and their Web sites, including sample documents to illustrate their content. These documents have also been chosen to show the various perspectives on the issues identified in the first two chapters of this book. Additional relevant organization and issue-oriented Web sites are presented in Chapter 6. Due to space limitations, sample documents from those sites could not be presented here.

Alliance for Health Reform

http://www.allhealth.org/

We have included here a number of examples of the material available as issues and fact sheets. We have included fact sheets on a number of the most important health reform–related topics. These fact sheets provide key points on the issues and a link to additional information on the topic. These include The Uninsured, Children's Coverage, Employer-Sponsored Coverage, Individual Coverage, Medicaid, Medicare, Prescription Drugs, Health Care Costs, Chronic Care, Long-Term Care, and Managed Care. The first four of these provide specific facts about aspects of insurance coverage and the lack of such. The next two provide this group's explanation of the two most important and long-standing programs to provide health insurance through government programs. Three of the sheets focus on some current issues in healthcare costs, and the last two focus on two more specialized issues of healthcare reform: long-term care and managed care.

The Uninsured: Key Facts

- In 2001, 41.2 million Americans, or 14.6 percent of the population, were uninsured for the entire year, according to the U.S. Census Bureau.
- In 2001, 10 percent of whites, 19 percent of blacks, and 33 percent of Hispanics were uninsured for the full year.
- More than 8 out of 10 of those who lack insurance are in working families.
- Of the nonelderly uninsured in 2000, nearly two-thirds (64 percent) lived on incomes below 200 percent of the federal poverty level for that year, or $28,300 for a family of three.
- In 2001, young adults (ages 18–24) were less likely than other age groups to have health insurance coverage. Twenty-eight percent of young adults were uninsured, compared with 16.7 percent of those ages 25–64 and less than 1 percent of those 65 years and older (due to widespread Medicare coverage for the elderly).
- The uninsured are more likely to experience avoidable hospitalizations and more likely to die during hospitalizations than those with health coverage.

- Uninsured adults were three times as likely as insured adults to have gone without a needed doctor visit, not filled a prescription, or not followed up on a recommended medical test or treatment in the past year because of an inability to pay (49 percent vs. 18 percent).

Children's Coverage: Key Facts

- Some 8.5 million children under the age of 18 were uninsured for all of 2001, or 11.7 percent of all children under the age of 18.
- Hispanic children were more than three times as likely as white, non-Hispanic children to be uninsured. Nearly 24.1 percent of Hispanic children lacked health insurance, compared to 7.4 percent of white, 13.9 percent of Black, and 11.7 percent of Asian and Pacific Islander children.
- Among the poor, 21.3 percent of children were uninsured during 2001.
- Estimates in 2000 suggested that 63 percent of uninsured children were low-income and eligible for Medicaid or the State Children's Health Insurance Program (SCHIP), but were not enrolled.
- Sixty-four percent of children are covered through a parent's employer.
- About 4.6 million children were enrolled in SCHIP at some point during fiscal year 2001, up from the 3.3 million in 2000.
- Medicaid covered more than one in four children at some point during 2002—23.9 million children under the age of 19.
- Uninsured kids are five times more likely to use the emergency room as a regular source of care than children with coverage.

Employer-Sponsored Coverage: Key Facts

- About 177 million Americans—62.6 percent of the population—had health coverage through an employer in 2001.
- The average monthly premium for health insurance in 2002 was $255 for an individual and $663 for a family.

The worker's share averaged $38 for individual coverage and $174 for family coverage.

- Premium costs rose 12.7 percent for the 12 months ending in spring 2002, compared with a 1.6 percent rise in general inflation and a 3.4 percent rise in wages.
- Just 55 percent of the smallest firms (three to nine workers) offered health insurance in 2002, compared with 99 percent of large companies (200 or more workers).
- Some 45 percent of low-wage workers (those earning $7 an hour or less) are not offered coverage on the job.
- Of low-wage workers who are offered coverage, 76 percent take it, even though most must pay a share of the premium. Of those declining coverage, more than half have coverage elsewhere, such as through a spouse's policy.
- Among higher-wage workers (those earning $15 an hour or more), 96 percent are offered coverage on the job. Some 94 percent of these eligible workers take the coverage.
- About two-thirds of current workers with health insurance would be guaranteed the right to continue their coverage under federal law if they were laid off. They would have to pay the costs of the entire premium.
- Five out of six workers who were offered health benefits in 2002 (84 percent) participated.

Individual Coverage: Key Facts

- About 16 million people, or 6.7 percent of those between the ages of 19 and 64, were covered by an individual health insurance policy in 1999. An individual policy is obtained in the private market to cover an individual or single family, and is not part of group coverage offered by an employer or government program.
- In all but five states, individuals or families buying insurance on their own can be charged higher premiums, or denied coverage, if they have health problems. The five exceptions are New Jersey, New York, Maine, New Hampshire, and Vermont.

- Federal law requires insurance companies to sell policies to anyone who has had at least 18 months of continuous coverage and is moving from a group policy to the individual market. There are no federal restrictions on how much companies may charge for coverage in such cases, although some states have set limits.
- High-risk pools existed in 30 states as of mid-2002, mostly for persons with big health care needs and no access to on-the-job coverage. Enrollment in all high-risk pools totaled about 105,000 in 1999. High-risk pools allow individuals with health problems, who can't afford or get coverage through private insurers, to obtain subsidized health insurance through the state.
- Many proposals to reduce the number of Americans without health insurance would subsidize coverage in the individual market, often through federal tax credits.

Medicaid: Key Facts

- Medicaid covered 44 million people at some time during 2000, including 22.6 million low-income children, 9.2 million low-income adults (ages 19 to 64), and 12 million low-income older persons or persons with disabilities. Over the course of a year, more people are covered by Medicaid than by Medicare.
- Medicaid spending is estimated to have accelerated sharply for 2001, growing at a projected 11.5 percent rate, compared with an 8.5 percent rise in 2000.
- Medicaid expenditures are expected to total $280 billion in 2003—$159 billion from the federal government and $121 billion from the states.
- Medicaid's share of state general fund spending grew from 10.5 percent in 1991 to 14.7 percent in 2001.
- Medicaid spending by states is expected to grow more than three and a half times faster than state revenues for 2002.
- Children account for 51 percent of those enrolled in Medicaid, but services to them consume only 15 percent of the Medicaid budget. The elderly and disabled account for approximately 27 percent of

persons enrolled in Medicaid, but their services consume 67 percent of the budget.

- Medicaid paid for approximately 17 percent of all hospital and 17 percent of all prescription drug spending in the U.S. in 2000.
- Medicaid is the largest source of health care financing, public or private, for people with disabilities. Medicaid covers one in five people with a specific, chronic disability.

Medicare: Key Facts

- In 2001, Medicare covered 40.1 million people, including 34.4 million elderly Americans (99 percent of the elderly population) and 5.7 million people under age 65 with disabilities or end-stage renal disease (ESRD).
- Medicare spending was $240 billion in 2001, or 12 percent of the federal budget, and is projected to rise to $600 billion, or 25 percent of the federal budget, in 2025.
- The government spent an average of about $6,100 per Medicare beneficiary in 2001.
- In 1998, 6 percent of Medicare beneficiaries accounted for nearly one-half of total expenditures.
- Fifty-one percent of Medicare beneficiaries have incomes below $25,000.
- In 1999, Medicare managed care enrollment peaked at 6.3 million, or 16 percent of Medicare beneficiaries, and declined to 5 million, or 12 percent, as of July 1, 2002.
- Thirty-eight percent of Medicare beneficiaries lacked prescription drug coverage in the fall of 1999.

Prescription Drugs: Key Facts

- Thirty-two new drugs and treatments were approved in 2001 by the Food and Drug Administration for conditions like HIV/AIDS, arthritis, cancer, Alzheimer's disease, heart disease, and schizophrenia.
- In 1999, doctors prescribed 146 drugs for every 100 visits, compared with 109 drugs per 100 visits in 1985.
- The average person had 10.3 prescriptions filled in 2000, compared with 8.3 five years earlier.

- The average price of a prescription from a retail pharmacy rose 10 percent in 2001, climbing to $49.84, from $45.27 the year before.
- Generic drugs accounted for 45 percent of prescriptions filled in 2001, but just 8 percent of dollars spent.
- Some 42 percent of uninsured adults who needed medications for high blood pressure were not taking them, compared with 25 percent of insured adults.
- Medicare beneficiaries are 14 percent of the U.S. population, but account for 43 percent of pharmaceutical prescriptions.
- People over 65 spent an average of $706 on drugs in 1999, or about 2.7 percent of their household spending, compared with $370 for all consumers, or 1 percent of household spending.
- Medicare beneficiaries with drug coverage used an average of 24 prescriptions in 1998, compared with 17 for Medicare beneficiaries without coverage. Beneficiaries in poor health who had drug coverage used 42 medications, compared with 27 for uninsured people in poor health who lacked drug coverage.

Health Care Costs: Key Facts

- Total national health care spending reached $1.3 trillion in 2000, or 13.2 percent of the nation's gross domestic product. Health care spending is projected to reach $2.6 trillion in 2010, an estimated 16.8 percent of the GDP.
- Total national spending on health care climbed 6.9 percent during 2000, marking the greatest one-year increase since 1993.
- Health care spending per capita rose 10 percent during 2001.
- Prescription drug costs have climbed dramatically over the past few years, increasing 18 percent in 2000 and 17 percent in 2001.
- In 2000, hospital costs rose 5.1 percent to $412 billion, the first one-year increase above the 4 percent level since 1993.
- Overall hospital spending increased 12 percent in 2001.

- Health insurance premiums for employers rose 11 percent in 2001, the largest increase since 1992. The increase in 2002 was 12.7 percent.
- Health maintenance organizations (HMOs) serving members of the California Public Employees' Retirement System (CalPERS), a large state employee benefit program, have negotiated premium hikes averaging 25 percent for 2003.

Chronic Care: Key Facts

- There are 125 million people with chronic conditions, a figure expected to rise to 171 million by 2030.
- Thirty-seven percent of all working-age Americans have at least one chronic health condition.
- The treatment of chronic conditions, combined with lost productivity, costs our society more than $650 billion a year.
- Average spending for a person with a chronic condition is $6,032 a year and can go as high as $16,000 a year if the individual needs help with the activities of daily living.
- Only one in four people with high blood pressure receive any treatment for this condition.
- Twenty percent of Medicare beneficiaries have five or more chronic conditions, and they account for two-thirds of Medicare spending.
- Asthma is the number one cause of school absences due to chronic conditions, with an average of 7.3 school days missed annually per student. The cost of care for asthma sufferers totals $7.5 billion a year.

Long-Term Care: Key Facts

- Of the estimated 13 million Americans needing long-term care, about 56 percent are over the age of 65.
- About 1.6 million people with long-term care needs reside in nursing homes.
- A year's stay in a nursing home costs roughly $50,000, and the average nursing home stay is about two and one-half years. The average annual cost for hiring someone to provide care at home is about $15,000.

- Medicare pays for virtually no custodial nursing home care.
- Six of every 10 Americans who reach age 65 eventually need some long-term care services.
- The average age of a nursing home resident is 84, and 74 percent of these residents are women.

Managed Care: Key Facts

- In 2001, 93 percent of Americans with health coverage were in managed care plans, compared with 54 percent in 1993.
- Preferred provider plans have become the dominant form of managed care, covering 48 percent of workers with health coverage in 2001, up from 16 percent in 1988.
- The percentage of Medicare beneficiaries enrolled in managed care peaked from 1998 to 2000 at 16 percent, up from 4 percent in 1992. That share dropped to 12 percent in July 2002.
- Medicaid enrollees in managed care rose to 57 percent in 2001, from 9 percent in 1990.
- Forty-two states have set up independent panels to review coverage decisions by managed care companies.

Center for Studying Health System Change

http://www.hschange.org/

The most recent reports the center has available on its Web site are cataloged in Tables 5.10 and 5.11, taken directly from the Web site.

We have included more details on two topics covered by this group. One document is an example of the tracking reports that the center produces, and the other is an example of an issue brief. The tracking report "So Much to Do, So Little Time: Physician Capacity Constraints, 1997–2001" deals with the important health policy issues of availability of physicians and their ability to manage the amount of work that needs to be done within the healthcare delivery system on an aggregate level. The second selection is an example of an issue brief. This particular brief uses the HSC data obtained from their project-site visits to discuss some particular healthcare cost and access issues.

TABLE 5.10
HSC Data Bulletins

Title	Date
Aging Plays Limited Role in Health Care Cost Trends	September 2002
Tracking Health Care Costs	September 2002
Tracking Health Care Costs	September 2001
Tracking Health Care Costs	November 2000
Some Communities Make Progress in Reducing Children's Uninsurance	October 2000
Who Is Likely to Switch Health Plans?	July 2000
Patients Concerned About Insurer Influences	June 2000
Why People Change Their Health Care Providers	May 2000

Source: Center for Studying Health System Change. http://www.hschange.org/index.cgi?func=pubs&what=1.
Accessed on January 27, 2003.

TABLE 5.11
HSC Tracking Reports

Title	Date
Back in the Driver's Seat: Specialists Regaining Autonomy	January 2003
Mounting Pressures: Physicians Serving Medicaid Patients and the Uninsured, 1997–2001	December 2002
Kinder and Gentler: Physicians and Managed Care, 1997–2001	November 2002
Working Families' Health Insurance Coverage, 1997–2001	August 2002
Who Do You Trust? Americans' Perspectives on Health Care, 1997–2001	August 2002
The Insurance Gap and Minority Health Care, 1997–2001	June 2002
Treading Water: Americans' Access to Needed Medical Care, 1997–2001	March 2002

Source: Center for Studying Health System Change. http://www.hschange.org/index.cgi?func=pubs&what=15.
Accessed on January 27, 2003.

So Much to Do, So Little Time: Physician Capacity Constraints, 1997–2001

Tracking Report No. 8
May 2003
Sally Trude

Signs of tightened physician capacity[1]—or physicians' ability to provide services relative to demand—appeared between 1997 and 2001, according to a study by the Center for Studying Health System Change (HSC). Patients waited longer for appointments, and more physicians reported having inadequate time with patients. Despite signs of tightened physician capacity, the supply of physicians grew modestly, the proportion of physicians working with nurse practitioners and other caregivers increased and doctors spent more time in direct patient care. This seeming contradiction emerged as the retreat from tightly managed care gave patients freedom to seek more care without substantial out-of-pocket cost increases. Current physician capacity constraints may ease if higher out-of-pocket costs prompt patients to seek less care.

Physician Supply Grows

The number of physicians in the United States continued to increase between 1995 and 2000, from 260 to 276 physicians per 100,000 people.[2] However, debates about a potential physician shortage have re-emerged.

As the practice of medicine changes rapidly and becomes increasingly complex, physicians have more diagnostic and treatment options for a larger pool of patients. Medical advances have transformed once terminal diseases—for example, many types of cancer—into chronic conditions that physicians must manage long term. Increased treatment capabilities may be causing physicians to shift how they spend time as they provide and interpret more diagnostic information and discuss results and treatment options with their patients and other physicians.

The current transition in the health care marketplace away from tight health plan restrictions also may have sparked temporary capacity constraints for physician services, complicating the debate about a potential physician shortage.

Physicians Spend More Time on Patient Care

Physicians spent more time in direct patient care between 1997 and 2001, but they worked fewer hours overall, according to the HSC Community Tracking Study Physician Survey. The time physicians spent in direct patient care grew from 44.7 hours a week in 1997 to 46.6 hours in 2001, while their average medically related work week fell from 55.5 hours to 54.4 hours during the same period (*see Table 1*). Overall, the proportion of time physicians spent in direct patient care activities increased from 81 percent in 1997 to 86 percent in 2001.

Medically related activities include time spent on administrative tasks, professional activities and direct patient care but exclude time spent on call when not actually working. Direct care of patients includes face-to-face contact with patients, as well as patient record-keeping and office work, travel time to see patients and communication with physicians, hospitals, pharmacies and others on patients' behalf.

Constrained physician capacity also may be affecting physicians' willingness to accept new patients. A growing proportion of physicians no longer accepts all new Medicare and privately insured patients, possibly because physicians face more patients seeking care and growing time pressures. The proportion of physicians accepting all new Medicare patients fell from 73 percent in 1997 to 69 percent in 2001, while the proportion of physicians accepting all new privately insured patients fell from 70.8 percent to 68.2 percent over the same period.

At the same time, more physician practices employed physician assistants, nurse practitioners, nurse midwives and clinical nurse specialists. The proportion of physicians in noninstitutional practice settings who worked with these caregivers increased from 40 percent in 1997 to 48 percent in 2001 (*see Figure 1*). The trend was most noticeable for group practices of three or more physicians, where the proportion employing nonphysician caregivers grew from 53 percent in 1997 to 66 percent in 2001.

Despite spending more time in direct patient care, a growing proportion of physicians reported having inadequate time with their patients.

More People Saw Doctors

The proportion of Americans who saw a physician at least once during the year grew slightly between 1997 and 2001, from 77 percent to 78 percent. Although slightly more people saw a doctor, and physicians spent more time in direct patient care, the average number of doctor visits per person remained constant.

Between 1997 and 2001, people had an average of 3.8 physician office visits a year. Practices' employment of nonphysician practitioners did not boost the average number of office visits per person, and the average number of office visits to either a physician or nurse practitioner remained unchanged— about four a year. Yet, more people reported seeing a nurse practitioner at least once during the year, with the proportion rising from 12 percent in 1997 to 15 percent in 2001.

Since the average number of office visits to either a physician or nurse practitioner was constant between 1997 and 2001, a possible explanation for the increase in people seeing a

FIGURE 1
Physicians in Practices[a] with Allied Health Professionals,[b] by Type of Practice

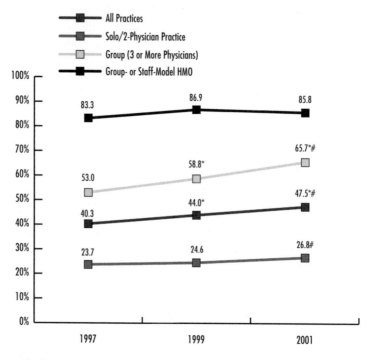

a. Practices in noninstitutional settings.
b. Includes physician assistants, nurse practitioners, nurse midwives, and clinical nurse specialists.
*Change from previous survey is statistically significant at p < .05.
#Change from 1997–2001 is statistically significant at p < .05.
Source: HSC Community Tracking Study Physician Survey.

TABLE 1
Physician Time Spent in Medically Related Activity and Direct Patient Care

	1997	1999	2001
Medically related: Average weekly hours	55.5	54.5[a]	54.4[b]
Direct patient care: Average weekly hours	44.7	44.7	46.6[b]
Percent of time in direct patient care	81.0	82.6	86.3[a, b]

[a]Change from previous survey is statistically significant at p < .05.
[b]Change from 1997–2001 is statistically significant at p < .05.
Source: HSC Community Tracking Study Physician Survey.

nurse practitioner is that more patients are seeing both a physician and a nurse practitioner during the same visit.

Where Does All the Time Go?

Despite spending more time in direct patient care, a growing proportion of physicians reported having inadequate time with their patients. When asked to agree or disagree with the statement, "I have adequate time to spend with my patients during office hours," 34 percent disagreed in 2001, compared with 28 percent in 1997 (*see Figure 2*). Other research, however, shows that time physicians spend face to face with patients did not change during the same period.[3]

Medical advances mean more treatment options are available to more patients. People are living longer with chronic illnesses that may require more complex coordination with other caregivers. With more diagnostic and treatment options available, physicians' increased time in direct patient care may reflect more time spent on patient care activities other than face-to-face visits with patients.

A growing list of recommended preventive services also may be consuming primary care physicians' time with patients. A recent study[4] estimated that if doctors followed all government recommendations aimed at preventing disease and injury, they would spend more than seven hours a day on the standards. Physicians may be frustrated by having too much to discuss with their patients in too little time.

Another indication of strained physician capacity is the growing proportion of people who did not get or postponed needed care because they could not get a timely appointment. In 2001, 5 percent of Americans did not get or postponed care because they couldn't get an appointment soon enough, compared with 3.4 percent in 1997.

Less-restrictive managed care practices and broader provider networks likely have made it easier for patients to see the physician of their choice. More patients can now bypass gatekeepers and preauthorization requirements when seeing specialists. Moreover, in 2001, because of the tight labor market, employers were reluctant to pass the rising costs of health insurance on to their workers and only made small increases to copayments and deductibles.

People may be receiving more care as a result of fewer restrictions and no substantial out-of-pocket cost increase. Without

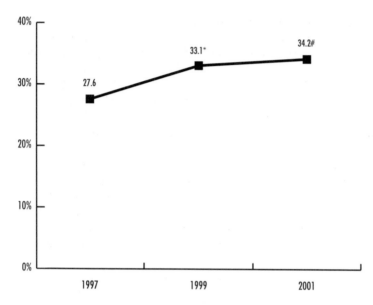

FIGURE 2
Physicians Reporting Inadequate Time with Patients

*Change from previous survey is statistically significant at p < .05.
#Change from 1997–2001 is statistically significant at p < .05.
Source: HSC Community Tracking Study Physician Survey.

a significant expansion in physician capacity, fewer managed care restrictions may have led to longer waits for appointments. However, as consumers must pay more out of pocket at the doctor's office, current capacity constraints may ease.

More Specialty Referrals

A growing proportion of primary care physicians reported referring more patients to specialists. In 2001, about one in four primary care physicians said they had referred more patients to specialists in the past two years, compared with less than one in five physicians in 1997 (*see Table 2*). Over this same period, managed care plans lifted many of the restrictions they had imposed on access to specialists, which likely accounts for some of the increase in referrals.

Yet, the proportion of primary care physicians who reported problems arranging referrals to specialists also grew slightly. Physicians were asked whether they were always, almost always, frequently, sometimes, rarely or never able to obtain referrals to high-quality specialists. Physicians were considered to have problems obtaining referrals if they reported "sometimes, rarely or never." Between 1997 and 2001, the proportion of primary care physicians reporting problems arranging specialty referrals increased from 4.8 percent to 7.2 percent. In contrast, the proportion of medical specialists who reported problems stayed about the same, while the proportion of surgical specialists who reported problems fell.

Waiting times for an appointment with a specialist grew between 1997 and 2001, but waiting times for primary care physicians remained unchanged. Half of all patients seeing a specialist for a specific illness waited 8.1 days or more in 2001, compared with 6.6 days or more in 1997. Half of all patients seeking an appointment with a primary care physician for a specific illness waited about a day.

Changes in specialists' willingness to accept all new patients regardless of their insurance coverage depended on the physician's specialty. Surgical specialists' willingness to accept all new Medicare, Medicaid and privately insured patients declined from 51 percent to 45 percent between 1997 and 2001. In contrast, a growing proportion of medical specialists accepted all new patients, while there was no change in the proportion of primary care physicians who accepted all new patients.

TABLE 2
Referrals to Specialists

	1997	1999	2001
Primary care physicians reporting increased referrals to specialists over the last two years	17.8%	21.6%[a]	25.5%[b]
Reporting problems obtaining referral to specialists			
Primary care physicians	4.8	4.6	7.2[a, b]
Medical specialists	10.8	11.3	10.2
Surgical specialists	12.2	12.2	7.8[a, b]

[a]Change from previous survey is statistically significant at $p < .05$.
[b]Change from 1997–2001 is statistically significant at $p < .05$.
Source: HSC Community Tracking Study Physician Survey.

The Shifting Marketplace

Revived debates about the adequacy of physician supply are occurring during an imbalance between patients seeking medical care and physician capacity. Yet, people on both sides of the debate agree that physician supply decisions should reflect long-term needs and not temporary fluctuations and imbalances in the availability of physician services.[5]

Currently, the U.S. health care marketplace is in transition from managed care restrictions such as gatekeeping and preauthorization to increased cost sharing for those who seek care. Although fewer managed care restrictions may have prompted people to seek more care and physicians to provide more care, physician capacity constraints may ease if people seek less care when faced with higher out-of-pocket costs.

The relative prominence of primary and specialty care may shift over time as well. When managed care plans' use of primary care physicians as gatekeepers swept the country in the early 1990s, the emphasis shifted away from specialist care to primary care.[6] As the number of people in tightly managed care increased, use of specialists was expected to fall. Estimates based on specialist-to-patient ratios in health maintenance organizations forecast a serious oversupply of specialists.[7] With fewer managed care restrictions limiting access to specialists, more people may seek specialist care, either directly or through their primary caregiver, but higher out-of-pocket costs may temper how often they seek specialty care.

Data Source

This Tracking Report presents findings from the HSC Community Tracking Study Physician Survey, a nationally representative telephone survey of physicians involved in direct patient care in the continental United States conducted in 1996–97, 1998–99 and 2000–01. For discussion and presentation, we refer to a single calendar year of the survey (1997, 1999 and 2001). The sample of physicians was drawn from the American Medical Association and the American Osteopathic Association master files and included active, nonfederal, office- and hospital-based physicians who spent at least 20 hours per week in direct patient care. Residents and fellows were excluded. Each round of the survey contains information on about 12,000 physicians, and the response rates ranged from 59 percent to 65 percent.

Notes

1. Physician capacity depends on a range of factors, including physician supply, the amount of time physicians are willing to devote to patient care, the mix of types of physicians and patients' demand for physician services.

2. Salsburg, Edward S., and Gaetano J. Forte, "Trends in the Physician Workforce, 1980–2000,"*Health Affairs,* Vol. 21, No. 5 (September/October 2002).

3. Mechanic, David, Donna D. McAlpine and Marsha Rosenthal, "Are Patients' Office Visits with Physicians Getting Shorter?" *The New England Journal of Medicine,* Vol. 344, No. 3 (Jan. 18, 2001).

4. Yarnall, Kimberly S. H., et al., "Primary Care: Is There Enough Time for Prevention?" *American Journal of Public Health,* Vol. 93, No. 4 (April 2003).

5. Cooper, Richard A., et al., "Economic and Demographic Trends Signal an Impending Physician Shortage," *Health Affairs,* Vol. 21, No. 1 (January/February 2002).

6. Grumbach, Kevin, "Fighting Hand to Hand Over Physician Workforce Policy," *Health Affairs,* Vol. 21, No. 5 (September/October 2002).

7. Weiner, Jonathan P., "Forecasting the Effects of Health Reform on U.S. Physician Workforce Requirement: Evidence from HMO Staffing Patterns," *Journal of the American Medical Association,* Vol. 272, No. 3 (July 20, 1994).

TRACKING REPORTS are published by the Center for Studying Health System Change. President: Paul B. Ginsburg Director of Public Affairs: Richard Sorian Editor: The Stein Group. Contact HSC at: 600 Maryland Avenue SW, Suite 550, Washington, DC 20024–2512 Tel: (202) 554–7549 (for publication information) Tel: (202) 484–5261 (for general HSC information) Fax: (202) 484–9258, *www.hschange.org.*

Source: Center for Studying Health System Change. http://www. hschange.org/CONTENT/556/. Accessed on August 20, 2003.

Health Care Cost and Access Problems Intensify

Initial Findings From HSC's Recent Site Visits
Issue Brief No. 63
May 2003
Cara S. Lesser, Paul B. Ginsburg

[Note: Only the first half of this report is included below.]

More detailed information on survey methodology can be found at www.hschange.org.

Continued high-cost trends are threatening the affordability of health insurance and many consumers' access to care. Early findings from the Center for Studying Health System Change's (HSC) 2002–03 site visits to 12 nationally representative communities show the retreat from tightly managed care continues to shape local health care markets. Employers are aggressively shifting higher health costs to workers, and absent tight managed care controls to limit the use of care and slow payment rate increases, hospitals and physicians in many markets are competing fiercely for profitable specialty services. These developments have sparked growing skepticism about the potential for market-led solutions to the cost, quality and access problems facing the health care system today.

Déjà Vu All Over Again

Two years ago, new cost and access problems emerged in the U.S. health care system as managed care lost its bite in the wake of a powerful consumer backlash. Health plans responded to consumer demand for broad choice of doctors and hospitals and loosened restrictions on care. Fewer restrictions on care led to higher utilization and taxed the capacity of many hospitals and physicians to meet demand. With broad provider networks and tighter capacity the norm, plans lost leverage over providers to negotiate price discounts—a key element in lower health cost trends throughout much of the 1990s. Facing rising premiums and reduced profits, some employers began to increase patient cost sharing in a bid to control health benefit outlays.

Along with higher costs, consumers confronted new barriers to care. Providers' greater clout sparked contract showdowns between prominent hospitals or physician groups and health plans, jeopardizing continuity of care for patients. Hospital capacity problems emerged for the first time in decades, causing emergency department diversions and endangering patients' access to timely care. Competition for high-margin specialty services, especially cardiac, cancer and orthopedic care, heated up among hospitals and physicians, prompting some providers to expand capacity for select profitable services rather than address broader capacity problems. Indeed, the aggressive copycat behavior and one-upmanship observed in many markets suggested a new medical arms race was underway.

Over the past two years, these trends have intensified. Higher cost sharing is widespread, affecting more employees and a greater number of services. Traditional strategies for managing care have continued to lose ground, and providers have stepped up expansion of lucrative specialty services, escalating concerns about costs and the implications of possible excess capacity in some areas. At the same time, many states face substantial budget shortfalls, prompting some immediate cuts in public health insurance programs and proposals for deeper cuts.

Access at a Cost: A New Deal for Employees

With the slow economy and three consecutive years of double-digit health insurance premium increases cutting into firms' bottom lines, employers are moving more aggressively to shift more health costs to workers. In some respects, this confluence of events recalls the early 1990s when employers struggled with rapidly rising premiums during an economic downturn and responded by aggressively shifting health benefit offerings to tightly managed care.

However, there are some key differences today. While labor markets have loosened since the late 1990s, they are not as severely depressed as a decade ago. The current 6 percent national unemployment rate is not high by historical standards, so employers are still somewhat cautious in responding to rising health costs. In addition, there was a great deal of optimism in the early 1990s about managed care and integrated delivery as an effective strategy to control rising health care costs and rationalize the health care system.

Today, a more modest vision is emerging as employers pin their hopes on the fledgling consumerism movement in health care to help rein in costs. The price and quality information consumers will need to make informed choices about the trade-offs among costs, quality and accessibility of care are still lacking for the most part, making the idea of consumer-driven health care a long-term strategy at best. Furthermore, some question whether incentives can be made powerful enough to lead to substantial changes in behavior without being perceived as barriers to care.

In the meantime, more employers are increasing cost sharing than two years ago, and employers are applying this strategy to a broader scope of services. Some employers, especially unionized firms and public sector employers, for the first time are requiring employees to make up-front contributions to health insurance premiums. Employers that already required premium contributions are increasing copayments and deductibles. And, in many cases, employers are replacing copayments, or fixed-dollar payments, with coinsurance, where patients pay a percentage of the price for services. The end result: Employees are seeing more of their paycheck going to premiums and paying more out of pocket when they fill a prescription or see a doctor.

Indeed, employers and benefit consultants interviewed in the 12 sites comment that, under the premise that managed care would control costs, employers assumed a much larger proportion of their employees' health care costs over the past decade. They now hope to readjust employee expectations and significantly increase workers' share of costs. However, unlike the move to managed care in the early 1990s, there is less confidence this strategy will have significant, long-term effects on care utilization patterns and delivery system efficiency.

Health Plans Prosper, Managed Care Wanes

Most health plans are more profitable than they were two years ago, mainly because premium increases have exceeded medical cost trends and plans have exited unprofitable lines of business, such as Medicare and Medicaid. But they are still reeling from the vigorous managed care backlash, and without a strong mandate from employers to reintroduce aggressive cost-control measures, plans have few tools to control costs.

Broad provider networks are now the norm, leaving plans with little credible threat of excluding hospitals as a way to negotiate lower payment rates. Global capitation arrangements, where providers assumed total financial risk for patients' care in return for a fixed payment, have all but disappeared in most communities, and even primary care capitation has declined substantially, eliminating a key financial incentive for providers to control care utilization. Many plans have scaled back traditional utilization management techniques, such as prior authorization and primary care gate-keeping, and some have moved away from conventional disease management programs. Most plans continue to pursue case management for the small percentage of high-cost patients who account for a large share of health care services, but the effect of these efforts is still quite limited.

Preferred provider organizations (PPOs) have replaced health maintenance organization (HMOs) as the platform of choice for health plan products. Plans also are experimenting with new PPO or HMO designs that sort network providers into different tiers with varying cost-sharing requirements, and they are developing consumer-driven health plans, or high-deductible plans with a personal spending account.

For the most part, these products are still on the drawing board or have been introduced only recently, with few takers to date. Although employers are now more interested in these products, most remain skeptical and are reluctant to be the first to sign up. Tiered-network products have faced stiff resistance from hospitals, which question the methodology used to establish the tiers. In some cases, hospitals have refused to participate in tiered networks and, in other cases, have used their negotiating leverage and political influence to avoid placement in high-cost tiers, limiting plans' ability to establish different tiers.

Some plans are emphasizing more customized products, with combinations of different benefit packages and network configurations. For example, in Indianapolis and Cleveland, Anthem Blue Cross Blue Shield has introduced a product, called Anthem by Design, that offers a choice of benefit add-ons to a base insurance product. Anthem likens the approach to buying a car, where a customer can add upgrades to a base model. As with other new product designs, such as consumer-driven products and tiered networks, these features are intended to reduce costs without sacrificing the broad choice of providers demanded by consumers. Critics, however, contend that consumers do not have enough information to make meaningful choices among these options.

Some plans are experimenting with incentive-based provider payments as an alternative to capitation. Rather than placing providers at financial risk for overutilization of care, these payment schemes reward providers for meeting quality and efficiency standards by supplementing base compensation with a bonus payment. Plans are experimenting with this approach in advanced managed care markets, such as Boston and Orange County, as well as in smaller markets with less managed care experience, such as Indianapolis, Cleveland and Syracuse. While incentive payments are more attractive to providers than financial risk, it is unclear whether the payments will be significant enough to get providers' attention and affect practice patterns and care delivery.

The Commonwealth Fund

http://www.cmwf.org

An example of the issue briefs produced by this group is included here. It is "Covering the Uninsured: Prospects and Problems." This is a multipage review of issues connected with covering the uninsured that also includes a list of thirty-nine additional citations at the end of the brief. The brief reviews some of the most pertinent facts about the current state of health insurance coverage, prospects for coverage expansion, and barriers to coverage expansion.

Covering the Uninsured: Prospects and Problems

Juliette Cubanski, John F. Kennedy School of Government, and Janet Kline, Health Policy Specialist

Introduction: The Current Status of Health Insurance Coverage

Increasing the number of Americans with health insurance has been a recurrent focus of federal and state policymaking, and recent trends suggest that the issue continues to warrant legislative attention. The number of people without health insurance coverage in the United States increased in 2001, a reversal of two years of falling rates of uninsurance. According to the Census Bureau, an estimated 14.5 percent of the total population (41.2 million people) lacked health insurance for the entire year in 2001, up from 14.2 percent in 2000—an increase of 1.4 million people.[1] Insurance coverage varies by state of residence, with New Mexico and Texas having the highest average uninsured rates from 1999 to 2001 (23 percent) and Rhode Island and Minnesota the lowest (7.8 percent). Private employment-based insurance remains the primary source of insurance coverage for most Americans, but public programs such as Medicare, Medicaid, and the state Children's Health Insurance Program (CHIP) are an important source of coverage for millions of elderly and disabled individuals and low-income children and adults.

Gaps in private and public coverage leave many Americans without access to health insurance or with only limited coverage. Many workers do not have access to employment-based insurance because they cannot afford it or their employer does not offer it.[2] Coverage in the private, non-group insurance market has been limited because premiums are based on an individual's age and health status, and are substantially more expensive than group plans purchased by employers.[3,4] Medicaid and CHIP cover many low-income Americans, primarily children, but eligibility criteria and covered services for these programs vary across states, resulting in coverage disparities. In addition to gaps that leave millions without insurance, researchers estimate that about one-fifth of insured individuals are underinsured, meaning that they face limits on coverage or substantial financial barriers to receiving treatment if they become ill.[5] Overall, these limitations in public and private coverage are not new. Yet recent trends—such as rising health care costs that fuel growth in health insurance premiums, and higher unemployment rates linked to a weakened economy—could lead to an erosion of the modest coverage improvements seen at the end of the 1990s.

Who Are the Uninsured?

People without insurance cannot easily be categorized. Demographic factors such as age, race, and ethnicity, as well as socioeconomic and employment status, affect health insurance coverage rates. The poor and near-poor have the greatest risk of being uninsured, but the large majority of uninsured also come from working families.[6] Exhibit 1 presents rates of the uninsured in 2001 by selected characteristics.

Trends in Public and Private Coverage

In 2001, almost 200 million people had private health insurance coverage. The vast majority, 176.5 million people, had employer-sponsored coverage. Public programs covered 71.3 million people, including 38 million enrolled in Medicare, 31.6 million covered by Medicaid, 9.5 million with military health care (including care provided by the Veterans Administration), and 2.3 million covered by CHIP. (Coverage estimates by type of plan are not mutually exclusive, since people can have both public and private coverage as well as both Medicare and Medicaid.) Rates of employment-based coverage gradually increased in the mid- to late-1990s, fueled by a good economy, low unemployment, and slower growth in insurance

EXHIBIT 1

Rates of the Uninsured in 2001 by Selected Characteristics

Ethnicity

Ethnicity	Rate
White	13.6%
Black	19.0%
Asian	18.2%
Hispanic	33.2%

Work experience

Work experience	Rate
Worked during year	17.0%
Worked full-time	16.0%
Worked part-time	22.0%
Did not work	24.7%

Income

Income	Rate
Less than $25,000	23.3%
$25,000–$49,999	17.7%
$50,000–$74,999	11.3%
$75,000 or more	7.7%

Age

Age	Rate
Under 18 years	11.7%
18–24 years	28.1%
25–34 years	23.4%
35–44 years	16.1%
45–64 years	13.1%
65 years and older	0.8%

Source: U.S. Census Bureau, *Current Population Survey, 202 Annual Demographic Supplement*.

premiums.[7] Enrollment in Medicaid declined following welfare reform in 1996, but state efforts to increase outreach and expand eligibility helped to stabilize Medicaid coverage. The CHIP program, begun in 1997, increased insurance coverage among low-income children. In 1999 and 2000, these coverage trends resulted in a decrease in the total number of uninsured. However, recent trends in coverage and rising health care costs may threaten coverage improvements. As described below, premiums for employer-sponsored coverage are increasing and many employers pass on these rising costs to their employees. States are facing budget constraints that may lead to cuts in eligibility and benefits in public programs such as Medicaid and CHIP. Reflecting these trends, half of insured individuals are worried about not being able to afford insurance or having benefits cut back in the coming year.[8]

EMPLOYER-SPONSORED INSURANCE TRENDS

The percent of people covered by employer-sponsored insurance decreased in 2001, from 63.6 to 62.6 percent.[9] The declining rate of employer coverage has been accompanied by increasing premiums. Between spring 2001 and spring 2002, monthly premiums for employment-based coverage rose 12.7 percent, significantly faster than wage gains for non-supervisory workers (3.4 percent).[10] Between 2001 and 2002, the worker's share of the overall premium rose by 27 percent for single coverage (an average of $454 per year in total) and 16 percent more for family coverage (an average of $2,084 per year in total).[11] In 2001, the average annual cost to an employer was $3,060 for individual coverage and $7,954 for family coverage.[12]

With a 15 percent average increase in health care premiums projected for 2003, additional increases in employee contributions are likely to occur in the future.[13] A variety of surveys find that employers plan to deal with rising health care costs by increasing employees' share of premiums as well as other cost-sharing measures. An employer survey found that 78 percent of large firms (200 or more workers) plan to increase employee premium contributions in the future, up from 44 percent in 2000.[14] Forty percent of workers in January 2002 reported that they paid more for employer-sponsored coverage in 2001 than in the previous year.[15] Along with increasing the employee contribution for premiums, employers are adopting cost-sharing methods that increase employees' responsibility for decisions about care. These include raising costs for care received out-of-network and copayments for physician and hospital services and prescription drugs. One-third of working adults report higher deductibles or copayments or benefit reductions in 2001 compared with the previous year.[16]

Employers are also evaluating new health plan benefit designs, such as defined contribution and consumer-driven or consumer-directed plans. These insurance arrangements are designed to give workers more choice, flexibility, and control in making health care decisions.[17] In defined contribution plans, employers offer employees a fixed sum to pay for coverage on their own. The employee pays any insurance costs that exceed the employer's contribution. Approximately one-quarter of firms say it is likely they will adopt this approach in the next few years.[18] Consumer-driven plans combine a high-deductible, catastrophic insurance policy (i.e., a major medical plan) with a health reimbursement account (HRA). In this arrangement, a portion of the employer's insurance contribution is placed in a personal health account from which employees can draw to purchase health care services with tax-exempt dollars.[18, 19] In June 2002, the Department of Treasury issued a ruling that clarifies that HRAs must be funded solely by the employer and cannot be funded by salary reductions, defines HRAs as group health plans subject to the COBRA continuation requirements, and allows unused balances in HRAs to carry over from one year to the next.[20] These features could increase the appeal of consumer-driven plans. According to a recent survey, about 30 percent of large employers say they will offer a consumer-driven plan by 2003.[21]

Requiring workers to pay higher cost-sharing amounts at the time of use reverses the trend toward lower cost-sharing amounts that accompanied the shift from indemnity insurance to managed care (e.g., a shift from a $100 deductible and 20 percent coinsurance to $10 per visit copayments). Some might argue that such a shift is overdue, since insurance arrangements have tended to insulate consumers from the actual cost of care, which may increase consumption of marginally beneficial services. Some might also argue that this shift is timely because managed care restrictions on use, which accompanied the lower cost-sharing, have been relaxed in recent years—giving rise to the term "managed care lite." Giving employees more control over their health spending through the use of consumer-driven plans could make basic coverage more available and affordable, thereby increasing coverage and relieving employers of increasing cost pressures, but it could also mean that some workers will pay more in costs at the time of use than under their old policies. The degree to which this ultimately will shift costs to workers will depend to a great extent on the amount the employer contributes as the lump sum and the correlation of high spending across years; i.e., whether high spending in one year is offset by low spending in another, so that in the low-spending year the worker comes out ahead. Requiring workers to pay higher premiums for the same coverage may lead some employees to drop coverage and thus exacerbate the problem of the uninsured.

TRENDS IN PUBLIC COVERAGE: MEDICAID AND CHIP

Among the entire population, the percent covered by government insurance programs rose in 2001, from 24.7 to 25.3 percent. This increase was largely due to an increase in the rate of Medicaid coverage, from 10.6 percent in 2000 to 11.2 percent in 2001.[22] According to the Census Bureau, Medicaid covered 31.6 million people in 2001. Beneficiaries include low-income mothers and children, and elderly and disabled individuals. Congress enacted CHIP as part of the Balanced Budget Act of 1997, providing $20.3 billion in federal funds over five years for states to expand coverage to low-income uninsured children. Enrollment in CHIP grew slowly during the initial years, but as of the end of 2001, total enrollment exceeded three million children. If the downward trend in private employer-sponsored insurance coverage continues beyond 2001, further increases in public program enrollment are likely to occur, absent changes at the state level to limit coverage expansions in order to reduce expenditures.

Prospects for Coverage Expansions

Recent policy debates have emphasized targeted approaches to expanding coverage. Current proposals include increasing enrollment in existing public programs, establishing tax benefits for purchasing health insurance, and expanding coverage through public-private linkages.

PUBLIC PROGRAM CREATION AND EXPANSION

Some policymakers support expanding coverage by building on existing public programs or creating new state-based programs. Proponents of these strategies argue that increasing coverage can be most easily accomplished by expanding eligibility for existing programs. Opponents are concerned about the substitution of public coverage for private coverage, and concerned that such expansions create a larger and less desirable role for government given that the private market is the predominant source of coverage.

Despite these concerns, a number of states have increased enrollment in existing programs by raising income or age eligibility levels for Medicaid and CHIP beyond federal minimums, and opening enrollment to parents of children eligible for these programs. Section 1115 of the Social Security Act provides authority to the secretary of the Department of Health and Human Services (HHS) to waive statutory provisions of the federal law to permit demonstration programs that further Medicaid program goals. As of May 2002, 8.2 million individuals received coverage under Section 1115 waivers, accounting for nearly one-fifth of all Medicaid spending.[23] The Bush administration has also enhanced the flexibility of states to increase coverage in Medicaid and CHIP through the Health Insurance Flexibility and Accountability (HIFA) waiver initiative. Announced in August 2001, HIFA is targeted at populations with incomes below 200 percent of the federal poverty level ($17,720 for an individual in 2002). HIFA allows states to finance coverage expansions by reducing the cost of public coverage in ways not otherwise permitted, such as reducing benefits and increasing cost-sharing for certain groups.[24] Such flexibility is viewed as essential by some states facing budget shortfalls that nevertheless want to implement public program expansions.

Using waiver authority, a few states have taken steps to extend Medicaid or CHIP coverage to low-income parents whose children are eligible for these programs. Research suggests that by covering parents, states can also increase the extent to which uninsured children are enrolled in Medicaid and CHIP.[25, 26] In 1999, 11 states and the District of Columbia expanded coverage to parents through either Medicaid or a separate state-funded program.[27] As of October 2002, HHS had approved waivers to cover parents using Medicaid or CHIP funds in six states (three of which also implemented expansions in 1999).[28, 29] Some states have created programs that target uninsured adults, financed solely through non-federal sources. For example, Pennsylvania's Adult Basic program uses $76 million from the state's share of the national tobacco settlement to provide low-cost health insurance for uninsured individuals ages 19 to 64 with low incomes (below 200 percent of the federal poverty level). However, current economic conditions have reduced state tax revenues nationwide and placed competing demands on limited state funds. Thus, the prospects for covering a large number of uninsured people through such state-based programs may be limited in the foreseeable future.

ESTABLISHING TAX BENEFITS FOR HEALTH INSURANCE

Many policymakers favor expanding coverage by creating tax benefits that provide financial incentives for individuals or employers to purchase health insurance. Options include creating a refundable tax credit for all workers, expanding and permanently extending Archer medical savings accounts (MSAs), creating tax credits for small employers, and expanding tax benefits for the self-employed.[30] Proponents of tax benefit approaches argue that they give consumers greater choice and control over their health insurance arrangements, and that they address equity and efficiency problems in current law regarding tax benefits. Opponents argue that these approaches are unlikely to make much difference for people who do not now purchase insurance. A primary concern with the tax credit approach is that depending on the size of the credit, it might not benefit lower-income families who cannot afford to purchase insurance before the subsidy kicks in. Opponents also argue that tax benefit approaches could erode the employment-based system but leave consumers with inadequate and more costly alternatives.

The 107th Congress considered various tax benefit proposals. Proposals were made to expand and permanently extend the authorization for MSAs (set to expire December 31, 2003); to allow self-employed taxpayers to deduct 100 percent of the cost of their insurance beginning in 2002; to allow individuals to deduct 100 percent of their insurance premiums, regardless of whether they itemize; and to authorize a tax credit for small employers (2 to 50 employees). In his Fiscal Year 2003 budget, President Bush allocated $89 billion over 10 years to establish a refundable tax credit for individuals under age 65. Under this approach, people who purchase coverage in the individual market could reduce their federal tax payments by some or all of the amount spent for insurance. A refundable tax credit would enable low-income people to claim the credit even if they owed no taxes.

While most of these proposals were not enacted in the 107th Congress, a tax credit provision was included in trade legislation signed into law in August 2002. The Trade Act of 2002 (P.L. 107–210) provides $12 billion over 10 years for benefits to trade-displaced workers, including a refundable tax credit to cover 65 percent of the cost of health insurance premiums. Uninsured workers who lose their jobs due to increased importation could use the tax credit to purchase insurance through employer-sponsored coverage offered by their former employers (i.e., COBRA coverage), or through state-sponsored insurance purchasing pools and high-risk pools.

EXPANDING COVERAGE THROUGH PUBLIC-PRIVATE LINKAGES

Some policymakers have proposed to expand coverage by using public funds to subsidize the purchase of employer-sponsored insurance. Such an approach could assist low-income people who are offered coverage by their employer, but who cannot afford the employee share of the premium. Proponents of premium assistance, or "buy-in," programs argue that the combination of public funds with employer contributions lessens the strain on both public and private payers and potentially allows funds to cover more people. Building on employer coverage could also help increase coverage by avoiding the stigma associated with enrollment in public programs.

Under current law, states can create premium assistance programs through the Medicaid Health Insurance Premium Payment (HIPP) program or through CHIP.[31] The cost of the buy-in must be no higher than what the state would have paid to enroll the individual in the public program (the cost-effectiveness test). Establishment of premium assistance programs to date has been limited because states have found the cost-effectiveness test difficult to demonstrate and have had trouble identifying eligible people—those who are enrolled in public programs but who could access employer-sponsored coverage.[32] HIPP enrollment represents only 1 percent of states' total Medicaid program enrollment.[33] To date, seven states have received approval from HHS to develop premium assistance programs using CHIP funds.[34] Despite limited experience with premium assistance, the use of this strategy is likely to increase. The HIFA initiative strongly encourages states to integrate Medicaid and CHIP funds with funds for private health insurance, and relaxes the cost-effectiveness guidelines to facilitate this activity. According to HIFA guidelines, states are not required to adhere to the cost-effectiveness test, but must monitor total costs and ensure that they are not significantly higher than if "buy-in" participants were enrolled in public programs. With this flexibility, states have opportunities to use public funds to subsidize private coverage among the low-income uninsured, while keeping within budget limits.

Potential Barriers to Coverage Expansions

Policymakers face difficult challenges in dealing with the uninsured problem, some of which are due to the design of the insurance system and the nature of public and private coverage. For instance, loss of employment can lead to loss of insurance, but the unemployed are not automatically covered elsewhere.[35] For those who lack a source of employment-based or public coverage, the individual market is the only option. Yet, coverage in this market is unstable and often unobtainable, the result of high prices, medical underwriting practices, and a small risk pool.[36] Also, many uninsured people may be eligible for public programs but do not participate because of enrollment barriers, lack of awareness, or concerns about stigma.

As states implement eligibility expansions through Medicaid and CHIP that target people at higher income levels, policymakers are concerned about minimizing the extent to which public coverage substitutes for existing private coverage. Estimates of the magnitude of this substitution effect, known as "crowd out," vary.[37] A primary concern is that employers might reduce or drop benefits for employees because of the availability of public coverage. In their public program expansions, states have implemented measures to minimize crowd out, such as imposing premiums and establishing waiting periods after losing private coverage. Such policies may prevent crowd out but also may result in more limited enrollment among the uninsured. Other barriers to expanding coverage stem from more recent trends in health care. For the first time in more than a decade, per capita health care spending rose at a double-digit rate in 2001, increasing by 10 percent.[38] National health spending is expected to grow faster than the gross domestic product (GDP) for the rest of the decade, with the health share of GDP projected to rise from 13.2 percent in 2000 to 17.0 percent by 2011.[39] Thus, even if the uninsured rate does not increase significantly in the near future, health care cost growth makes any measures that would reduce the current uninsured population more expensive.

Conclusion

Incomplete insurance coverage has been a formidable problem for policymakers. Solutions, whether incremental or broader in scope, involve decisions about how to invest public funds. Reaching out to a broad spectrum of uninsured individuals could require a substantial investment of public and private dollars. Conversely, minimizing costs in the current constrained budget environment may mean restricting or limiting the target population for coverage expansions. The factors that currently exist—higher health care costs, increasing insurance premiums and cost-sharing amounts, unemployment growth, and state budget restrictions—suggest that making significant inroads in the uninsured population may be difficult in the foreseeable future.

EXHIBIT 2

Percent of People Without Health Insurance for the Entire Year by State: 3-Year Average, 1999–2001

State	Percent	State	Percent	State	Percent
United States—Total	14.5	Kentucky	13.0	Ohio	10.8
Alabama	13.2	Louisiana	19.7	Oklahoma	17.9
Alaska	17.7	Maine	10.7	Oregon	13.1
Arizona	18.4	Maryland	11.3	Pennsylvania	8.7
Arkansas	15.0	Massachusetts	8.7	Rhode Island	7.2
California	19.2	Michigan	9.9	South Carolina	13.3
Colorado	15.1	Minnesota	7.8	South Dakota	10.4
Connecticut	9.7	Mississippi	15.2	Tennessee	10.8
Delaware	9.5	Missouri	8.8	Texas	23.0
District of Columbia	13.6	Montana	16.0	Utah	13.6
Florida	17.8	Nebraska	9.6	Vermont	9.7
Georgia	15.3	Nevada	17.2	Virginia	11.9
Hawaii	9.7	New Hampshire	9.0	Washington	13.5
Idaho	16.5	New Jersey	12.5	West Virginia	14.2
Illinois	13.6	New Mexico	23.2	Wisconsin	8.5
Indiana	10.8	New York	15.8	Wyoming	15.6
Iowa	8.0	North Carolina	14.2		
Kansas	11.4	North Dakota	10.9		

Source: U.S. Census Bureau, *Current Population Survey,* 2002 Annual Demographic Supplement.

References

1. Robert J. Mills. *Health Insurance Coverage: 2001.* Current Population Reports P60-220. U.S. Census Bureau, September 2002.

2. Jeanne M. Lambrew. *How the Slowing U.S. Economy Threatens Employer-Based Health Insurance.* The Commonwealth Fund, November 2001.

3. Kaiser Commission on Medicaid and the Uninsured. *The Uninsured: A Primer.* Henry J. Kaiser Family Foundation, March 2002.

4. Jon Gabel, Kelley Dhont, and Jeremy Pickreign. *Are Tax Credits Alone the Solution to Affordable Health Insurance? Comparing Individual and Group Insurance Costs in 17 U.S. Markets.* The Commonwealth Fund, May 2002.

5. Kaiser Commission on Medicaid and the Uninsured. *Underinsured in America: Is Health Coverage Adequate?* Henry J. Kaiser Family Foundation, July 2002.

6. Kaiser Commission, *The Uninsured: A Primer,* March 2002.

7. John K. Iglehart, "Changing Health Insurance Trends," *New England Journal of Medicine* 347 (September 19, 2002): 956–62.

8. Kaiser Commission, *Underinsured in America,* July 2002.

9. Mills, *Health Insurance Coverage: 2001,* September 2002.

10. Iglehart, "Changing Health Insurance Trends," September 19, 2002.

11. Kaiser Family Foundation/Health Research and Educational Trust. *Employer Health Benefits: 2002 Summary of Findings.* Kaiser Family Foundation, September 2002.

12. Ibid.

13. Hewitt Associates. "Health Care Cost Increases Expected to Continue Double-Digit Pace in 2003." Press Release, October 14, 2002. Accessible at http://was.hewitt.com/hewitt/resource/newsroom/pressrel/2002/10-14-02.htm/, accessed October 21, 2002.

14. Kaiser/HRET. *Employer Health Benefits,* September 2002.

15. Jennifer Edwards et al. *The Erosion of Employer-Based Health Coverage and the Threat to Workers' Health Care.* The Commonwealth Fund Issue Brief, August 2002.

16. Ibid.

17. Hewitt Associates. "Health Care Cost Increases," October 14, 2002.

18. Kaiser/HRET. *Employer Health Benefits,* September 2002.

19. Iglehart, "Changing Health Insurance Trends," September 19, 2002.

20. The ruling specifies that maximum reimbursement amounts deposited by an employer in an employee's HRA in one year would be increased by any unused reimbursement amounts from previous years. The ruling is accessible at http://www.ustreas.gov/press/releases/docs/rev.rul.pdf/, accessed November 22, 2002.

21. Kathy Kristof, "New Health Care Plans May Not Be a Panacea." *Los Angeles Times,* August 25, 2002.

22. Mills, *Health Insurance Coverage: 2001,* September 2002.

23. Jennifer Ryan. *1115 Ways to Waive Medicaid and CHIP Rules.* National Health Policy Forum, Issue Brief No. 777, June 2002.

24. Jennifer Ryan. *Health Insurance Family Style: Public Approaches to Reaching the Uninsured.* National Health Policy Forum, Issue Brief No. 767, September 24, 2001.

25. Lisa Dubay and Genevieve Kenney. *Covering Parents Through Medicaid and CHIP: Potential Benefits to Low-Income Parents and Children.* Kaiser Commission on Medicaid and the Uninsured, October 2001.

26. Institute of Medicine. *Health Insurance Is a Family Matter.* Washington, D.C.: National Academies Press, 2002.

27. Dubay and Kenney, *Covering Parents,* October 2001.

28. Ryan, *Health Insurance Family Style,* September 24, 2001.

29. Centers for Medicare and Medicaid Services. State Children's Health Insurance Program (CHIP) Approved Section 1115 Demonstration Projects, October 7, 2002. Accessible at http://www.cms.gov/CHIP/1115waiv.pdf/, accessed November 4, 2002.

30. Medical savings accounts are personal savings accounts for unreimbursed medical expenses. They are used to pay for health care not covered by insurance, including deductibles and copayments. The formal name of MSAs is now Archer MSAs. The original MSA legislation (the Health Insurance Portability and Accountability Act of 1996, P.L. 104-191) authorized a limited number of MSAs under a demonstration beginning in 1997.

31. Ryan, *Health Insurance Family Style,* September 24, 2001.

32. Leslie Conwell and Ashley Short. *Premium Subsidies for Employer-Sponsored Health Coverage: An Emerging State and Local Strategy to Reach the Uninsured.* Center for Studying Health System Change, Issue Brief No. 47, December 2001.

33. Ryan, *Health Insurance Family Style,* September 24, 2001.

34. Ibid.

35. Lambrew, *How the Slowing U.S. Economy,* November 2001.

36. Office of the Assistant Secretary for Planning and Evaluation, Department of Health and Human Services. *Assessing the Individual Health Insurance Market in the Post-HIPAA Era: A Review of the Literature,* June 2001.

37. See, for instance, Richard Kronick and Todd Gilmer, "Insuring Low-Income Adults: Does Public Coverage Crowd Out Private?" *Health Affairs* 21 (January/February 2002): 225–37; David Cutler and John Gruber, "Does Public Insurance Crowd-Out Private Insurance?" *Quarterly Journal of Economics* 111 (2): 391–430; Linda Blumberg et al., "Did the Medicaid Expansions for Children Displace Private Insurance? An Analysis Using the SIPP," *Journal of Health Economics* 19 (1): 33–60.

38. Bradley Struck et al. "Tracking Health Care Costs: Growth Accelerates Again in 2001," *Health Affairs* Web Exclusive, September 25, 2002. W299–W310.

39. Alliance for Health Reform. *Health Care Costs & Health Coverage, August 2002.* August 21, 2003.

Families USA

http://www.familiesusa.org/html/about/about.htm

Two examples of Families USA materials are included here. One of these is "The President's Budget Shortchanges America's Health Care Needs." This brief report provides an overview of the budget proposals of 2003 and is an excellent example of the types of critiques this organization makes of the proposed programs for that year. Issues related to Medicare, prescription drugs, and Medicaid are included in the comments. The second report, "Nearly One Out of Three Non-Elderly Americans Were Uninsured for All or Part of 2001–2002," highlights a report it released detailing the increasing problem of uninsured Americans. Below are the press releases for these reports, with the full reports available at their site at no cost.

The President's Budget Shortchanges America's Health Care Needs

Bush's budget priorities don't add up to his State of the Union promises
Ron Pollack, executive director of Families USA, released the following statement today in response to President Bush's budget proposal:

"The budget released today by President Bush does not add up to the health care promises he made to the American people in his State of the Union address. The President's budget falls far short of the fiscal commitment needed to fulfill his promise of 'quality, affordable health [care] for all.'

"Even worse, the Administration's proposals to coerce seniors into HMOs and managed care plans, and its proposal to create a block grant in lieu of Medicaid coverage for millions of low-income families, will do considerable harm. These proposals will force seniors to lose their doctors and will cause many of the most vulnerable people to join the ranks of the uninsured.

Medicare and Prescription Drugs
"President Bush's budget includes $400 billion for both Medicare restructuring and prescription drug coverage over the next ten years. Unfortunately, $400 billion only covers a very meager

share of seniors' prescription drug costs, which are projected to total $2 trillion over the same ten-year period.

"The President's new proposal to force seniors into private health plans, as a condition for receiving prescription drug coverage, pressures seniors into choosing between the drug coverage they so desperately need and the doctors they have come to depend on.

"Private health plans participating in Medicare have a poor record serving seniors. They are unavailable in many rural communities, and they frequently leave communities that are deemed unprofitable. The private plans that continue to enroll seniors are, with each passing year, significantly increasing seniors' costs and decreasing the services offered.

"The coupling of prescription drug coverage with enrollment in HMOs and managed care plans will make it much more difficult to enact prescription drug coverage in this Congress. President Bush should not hold seniors' prescription drug coverage hostage to the achievement of his goal to privatize Medicare.

Medicaid

"The President's Medicaid budget represents a cruel hoax for three very important reasons. First, the President offers a slight increase in Medicaid funding in the first years, but then reduces such funding in the later years. Over the long term, this proposal would significantly reduce the federal aid needed to sustain Medicaid coverage for low-income families.

"Second, the President's proposal would establish ironclad caps in federal funding for health care to low-income families. As a result, when the economy turns sour, or health care costs skyrocket, or more people become uninsured, states will have a diminished capacity to meet their needs.

"Third, the President's proposal offers modest upfront money in a manner that is reminiscent of a loan shark. The modest upfront money comes attached with a heavy cost—less money in the long run and much less fiscal flexibility in future years. In effect, the Bush Administration is forcing cash-strapped states to buy into a very bad deal so that they can receive quick money now.

"The President's proposed block grant is similar to the failed proposal in 1995 by then-Speaker Newt Gingrich. This block grant will force states to ration care by limiting the number of people enrolled in Medicaid, reducing the services covered, and increasing the amount of money low-income people must pay.

Access
"Once again, the President included $89 billion over ten years in his budget for health tax credits. The tax credit proposed is far too small to make health coverage affordable for the low-wage workers targeted for this plan. It is like throwing a 10-foot rope to a person stuck in a 40-foot hole.

   "Also, in these tough economic times, the proposed tax credit offers no relief for many recently unemployed workers because the tax credit cannot be used to continue employer-based coverage through COBRA. Thus, this proposal does not reflect the President's promise to reduce the number of uninsured Americans."

   Families USA is the national organization for health care consumers. It is nonprofit and nonpartisan and advocates for high-quality, affordable health care for all Americans.

   Source: Families USA. http://www.familiesusa.org/site/PageServer?
pagename=PresidentsBudgetShortchange. Accessed on August 20, 2003.

Nearly One Out of Three Non-Elderly Americans Were Uninsured for All or Part of 2001–2002
New State-by-State Report Finds That 75 Million People Were Uninsured in Last Two Years, Most for Very Long Periods of Time

Families USA prepared a report for Cover the Uninsured Week (CTUW) that was released today by The Robert Wood Johnson Foundation as part of the kickoff for CTUW. The Families USA report, based on Census Bureau data, found that 74.7 million Americans under 65 years of age—almost one out of three (30.1 percent)—were uninsured at some point during 2001–2002. Almost two-thirds (65 percent) of these uninsured people were without health coverage for at least six months, and nearly one-quarter (24 percent) were uninsured throughout the two-year period.

The following is the statement of Ron Pollack, executive director of Families USA, concerning the report:

"The findings in this report should represent a sea change in the way we think about the uninsured. Now that almost one out of three non-elderly Americans experienced significant periods without health insurance, the uninsured problem is no longer simply an issue of altruism about other people, but it is also one of self-interest for us all.

"As the 75 million who were uninsured over the past two years reflect, working families are increasingly at risk of becoming uninsured—whether due to a pink slip from a job, unaffordable cost increases, or cutbacks in employer and public health coverage.

"With large and growing portions of the U.S. population becoming uninsured, we are moving towards a political tipping point that will require real and meaningful action to expand health coverage."

Source: Families USA. http://www.familiesusa.org/site/PageServer?pagename=nearly. Accessed on August 20, 2003.

Henry J. Kaiser Family Foundation

http://www.kff.org/

Two examples of portions of some of the Henry J. Kaiser reports are included here. One, "The Cost of Not Covering the Uninsured Project," is an excerpt from research conducted for the foundation on issues of the uninsured. The second is "Bush Administration Medicaid/SCHIP Proposal" and includes a discussion of issues related to President Bush's proposals concerning these two important publicly funded programs. This information was reprinted with permission of the Henry J. Kaiser Family Foundation. The Kaiser Family Foundation, based in Menlo Park, California, is a nonprofit, independent national healthcare philanthropy and is not associated with Kaiser Permanente or Kaiser Industries.

The Cost of Not Covering the Uninsured Project

June 2003

Much of the ongoing debate over ensuring health coverage for the over 40 million Americans who have no health insurance today revolves around the questions of how much it will cost and who ought to pay. The debate periodically stalls, perhaps in part, because the full benefits of universal coverage—particularly the economic benefits—to both the individual and the nation as a whole, have not yet been fully measured and discussed.

The Kaiser Family Foundation initiated The Cost of *Not* Covering the Uninsured project to explore what is known and what should be known about the costs society incurs when so many have no health insurance coverage. Under this initiative, we convened an expert advisory group that worked with staff of the Kaiser Commission on Medicaid and the Uninsured to plan and oversee new analyses and reports that would further the understanding of this critical issue.

This brief summarizes the initiative's first three analyses and reports, conducted by Jack Hadley, Ph.D. and John Holahan, Ph.D. of the Urban Institute. The project's advisory group was chaired by Robert Reischauer, President of the Urban Institute, and consisted of Sheila Burke, Arnold Epstein, Judy Feder, Uwe Reinhardt, Dorothy Rice, Earl Steinberg, Jim Tallon, and Marta Tienda.

Key Findings

- The uninsured receive less preventive care, are diagnosed at more advanced disease stages, and once diagnosed, tend to receive less therapeutic care and have higher mortality rates.
- A conservative estimate based on the full range of studies is that a reduction in mortality of 5–15% could be expected if the uninsured were to gain continuous health coverage.
- Better health would improve annual earnings by about 10–30 percent and would increase educational attainment.
- On average, the uninsured receive about half as much care as people who are insured all year. In 2001, persons uninsured for the full year used $1,253 per year in medical care compared to $2,484 for persons with private coverage for the full year.
- Total uncompensated care provided in 2001 was estimated to be $35 billion. The primary source of funding for uncompensated care is government, which

spent an estimated $30.6 billion for care of the uninsured, two thirds of which is federal.

- If insurance coverage were comparable to an "average" public health plan, estimated per person spending by people uninsured for any part of the year would rise by a little over 50%, increasing from $1,383 to $2,121. Under an "average" private health plan, spending would rise to $2,676.

- Expanding coverage to the entire uninsured population would increase spending by $34 billion under a public coverage standard and $69 billion under a private coverage standard. Including the $99 billion in medical care already used by the uninsured, the total cost of medical care used by the previously uninsured under universal coverage would range from $133 billion to $168 billion.

- The overall impact of universal coverage on total health care costs would be an increase of 3–6% in total health care spending in the U.S., less than the annual inflation in health care spending (8.7% in 2001) in the current health care system.

Source: Henry J. Kaiser Family Foundation. http://www.kff.org/content/2003/4118/4118.pdf. Accessed on August 20, 2003.

Medicaid and the Uninsured: Bush Administration Medicaid/SCHIP Proposal

[Note: Only the first part of this report is included below.]

May 2003

With states facing their worst fiscal crisis since World War II, the Medicaid program now is in a period of significant stress. In light of severe budget problems and rising Medicaid costs, states have called on the federal government for more help in paying for Medicaid and more flexibility over Medicaid funds. In response, some in Congress have put forth proposals to temporarily increase the share of Medicaid that is paid for by the federal government, while others have encouraged a reexamination of Medicaid's role in paying for long-term care and prescription drugs for seniors enrolled in Medicare.

In January of 2003, the Administration put forth a proposal to restructure Medicaid and SCHIP in ways that could fundamentally alter the two programs. The proposal, which is the subject of this policy brief, is now being considered on Capitol Hill and by a Taskforce established by the nation's Governors to develop and evaluate Medicaid reform proposals. It gives states the choice of remaining in the current Medicaid/SCHIP program or opting into a new system that combines increased flexibility over benefits and coverage with capped federal financing. The proposal gives states immediate financial incentives to opt for the new system, but federal funding would be reduced in later years. In states that take the option, the new system would end Medicaid as an entitlement program for many beneficiaries and eliminate open-ended federal financing. Although capped federal funding would increase over time by a specified trend factor, the combination of fewer rules over how the funds are used, repeal of matching requirements, and fixed federal allotments make the new structure essentially a block grant.

This policy brief begins with a brief overview of key challenges confronting the Medicaid program (Section I). It then provides a detailed explanation of what is known about the key elements of the Administration's proposal (Section II). The brief concludes with a discussion of the implications of the Administration's proposal (Section III).

I. Key Challenges Confronting Medicaid

Medicaid is the nation's major public financing program for providing health and long-term care coverage to over 50 million low-income Americans. . . . It plays a major role in the nation's health care system, paying for 17% of hospital care, 17% of prescription drug spending, and half of nursing home care. An entitlement to states and individuals, Medicaid provides open-ended federal matching funds to enable states to respond to unexpected changes in economic conditions, increases in poverty, rising health and long-term care costs, public health epidemics, and emergencies or disasters.

As a program financed jointly by the federal government and the states, Medicaid now is in a period of significant stress. States are facing their worst fiscal crisis since World War II due to dramatic declines in their revenues. Over the last two years state revenues have fallen faster and further than anyone predicted, creating state budget shortfalls of $49 billion this year and close to $70 billion for FY 2004. . . . The states' fiscal crisis is being driven by the economic downturn and outdated state tax structures, but also affects states' ability to finance their share of Medicaid costs, particularly given that Medicaid spending is growing relatively rapidly.

In fiscal year 2002, Medicaid spending grew 13 percent and this year it is expected to increase by 10 percent. The growth in the program is due in large part to the rapidly rising cost of providing prescription drugs and other health and long-term care services to elderly and disabled beneficiaries. . . . Of particular note is the cost to Medicaid of covering "dual enrollees," low-income seniors and disabled individuals who are enrolled in both Medicare and Medicaid. Although dual enrollees receive their basic health care benefits through Medicare, they use Medicaid to help with the cost of prescription drugs, long-term care and other services not generally covered by Medicare, as well as with Medicare premium and cost-sharing obligations. Many dual enrollees have particularly extensive health care needs and, as a result, they consume a disproportionately high share of Medicaid spending—a little under one-fifth of Medicaid enrollees also are enrolled in Medicare, but these dual enrollees consume more than a third of all Medicaid spending. . . .

Turning first to rainy day and tobacco settlement funds, states have tried to preserve Medicaid and keep the federal dollars in the program and their state economies. But as these sources have become depleted, states have had to turn to cuts in Medicaid. A recent KCMU survey found that 49 states were planning or taking action to reduce the growth in Medicaid spending. Nearly half of the states were turning to reducing benefits or limiting eligibility. . . .

In response to these fiscal pressures, states have called on the federal government for more help with the cost of operating Medicaid, particularly with the expense of providing prescription drugs and long-term care to Medicare beneficiaries also enrolled in Medicaid. They also have renewed long-standing calls for additional flexibility over how they use their Medicaid funds. The Administration's proposal . . . also is being considered by members of Congress and Governors as a vehicle for addressing the concerns of states.

Source: Henry J. Kaiser Family Foundation. http://www.kff.org/content/2003/4117/4117.pdf. Accessed on August 20, 2003.

Heritage Foundation

http://www.heritage.org/Research/HealthCare/index.cfm

The Heritage Foundation is a conservative think tank. Its Health Care Web page provides access to Heritage-sponsored reports on the healthcare system and health reform from a conservative viewpoint. An example of one of their reports is "Building a Better Medicare Program: The Senate Aging Committee's Focus on Patient Choice and Market Competition." This brief report summarizes testimony about reform to Medicare and focuses on demographic challenges, structural design issues, and cost control.

Building a Better Medicare Program: The Senate Aging Committee's Focus on Patient Choice and Market Competition

by Derek Hunter
WebMemo #279
May 22, 2003

The U.S. Senate Special Committee on Aging examined ways to strengthen and improve the Medicare program, the huge government health care program that insures 41 million senior and disabled citizens. The Special Committee, chaired by Sen. Larry Craig (R-ID) with Sen. John Breaux (D-LA) as the ranking minority member, held the hearing on May 6, 2003.

Three panelists testified on the value of patient choice and market competition:

1. Robert E. Moffit, Ph.D., director of the Center for Health Policy Studies at The Heritage Foundation;
2. Joseph R. Antos, Ph.D., health policy analyst at the American Enterprise Institute; and
3. Walton Francis, an economist and consultant on health policy.

The witnesses cited the record and experience of the Federal Employees Health Benefits Program (FEHBP), the health plan that covers 8.3 million federal workers including Members of Congress, federal retirees, and their families. Also testifying before the Senate panel was Abby Block, senior advisor for employee and family support policy with the U.S. Office of

Personnel Management (OPM), the government agency that administers the FEHBP.

Block outlined the flexible FEHBP structure and how it differs from the rigid Medicare program, where an act of Congress or a complicated administrative process is required to change or modify the health benefits package.

"While all participating plans offer a core set of benefits broadly outlined in statute, benefits vary among plans because there is no standard benefits package," Block told the Senate panel.

While Congress must approve new procedures and technologies in order for them to be covered by Medicare, the FEHBP offers competition among plans offering many sets of benefits so that members can choose what best suits their needs. Setting up a basic framework without micromanaging benefits, said Block, allows "OPM to focus on three key elements: policy design, contract negotiations, and contract administration including financial oversight."

The Demographic Challenge. Moffit questioned whether the existing Medicare structure was capable of absorbing the coming retirement of the baby-boom generation. "The central policy question facing Congress and the Administration" said Moffit, "is whether Medicare, as it exists today, can absorb the demographic shock of the baby-boom generation and continue to deliver high-quality medical care in an economically efficient fashion. I do not think that it can."

The Structural Design Problems. Francis called Medicare's design "obsolete," a "vintage 1960 design." Francis said that Medicare not only fails to cover prescription drugs, preventive care, dental costs, or care received abroad (with the exception of Canada and Mexico), but also "does not provide a catastrophic ceiling on costs even for those costs it covers." In sharp contrast, Francis argued, "None of these deficiencies affect the FEHBP. That program was also created vintage 1960, but it has painlessly evolved over time through the competitive, consumer-driven process that is its central feature."

The Record on Cost Control. Antos, a former Assistant Director of the Congressional Budget Office (CBO), addressed the issues of comparative cost between private-sector plans and Medicare, including recent research on the subject. Antos noted, "Medicare has been more successful than the private sector in constraining spending growth over the long term." Examining data over three decades, he further noted that "private insurance became *more generous* over that time period, covering a growing proportion of the total cost of health services. In 1970, private insurance paid for about 60 percent of the total private cost of hospital and physician services. By 1999, that had grown to 85 percent."

In conclusion, Antos said, "A Medicare reform modeled after FEHBP would provide both the incentive and the opportunity for seniors to choose health plans that best meet their needs." Echoing that view, Francis told the Senate panel that:

> The choice before the Congress ultimately is between these two models—consumer choice or detailed legislative and bureaucratic control. By good fortune we have as an example the successful performance of the consumer choice model in meeting the health insurance needs of 9 million employees and retirees. Surely we can use that model to aid in reforming the Medicare program.

Moffit likewise urged the Senate panel to examine the FEHBP model as a way to accommodate the needs of a large and diverse baby-boom generation that is set to start retiring in eight years.

Source: Heritage Foundation. http://www.heritage.org/Research/HealthCare/wm279.cfm. Accessed on August 21, 2003.

National Center for Policy Analysis

http://www.ncpa.org/

Many of the center's reports are more in-depth examinations of topics, rather than responses to a specific new proposal. An example of one of these is the report "Reforming Medicaid." Included here is the executive summary of this report, which focuses on a more comprehensive review of Medicaid, its past, variation by state, and special groups of Medicaid recipients (such as the disabled and those receiving long-term care).

Reforming Medicaid

by James R. Cantwell
U.S. House Committee on the Budget
Policy Report No. 197NCPA
August 1995, ISBN #1–56808–062-X

Executive Summary

While growth in private-sector health care spending has declined recently, spending on Medicaid, the federal-state health insurance program for the nation's poor, has continued to explode—growing at an average annual rate of 19.1 percent between 1990 and 1994. The Congressional Budget Office estimates that federal outlays for Medicaid will be $89.2 billion in 1995, and states will spend an additional $67.3 billion, for a total of $156.5 billion. Unless Congress reins in the growth of Medicaid, any attempt to balance the federal budget will be futile.

Both the Republican-led Congress and the Clinton administration have proposed budgets that call for reducing the rate of growth of Medicaid spending. The congressional plan, providing for less growth than the administration's plan, calls for giving Medicaid funds to each state in the form of a block grant. Block-granting the funds would allow the federal government to limit the financial exposure of taxpayers while giving states maximum flexibility to design a health care program that meets local needs.

Critics have charged that slowing the rate of growth of Medicaid spending would force states to reduce the number of people covered, reduce benefits, reduce payments to providers or some combination of these. However, six constructive steps described in this study could achieve Medicaid savings of $185.4 billion over seven years without any reduction in benefits for needy people.

- Changing incentives for recipients and providers through Medical Savings Accounts and/or managed care would produce $37.2 billion savings in acute care programs and $64 billion in long-term care.
- Enforcing estate recovery provisions would produce savings of $35 billion.
- Redirecting and capping "disproportionate share hospital" payments would produce savings of $13.9 billion.
- Reducing administrative costs would produce savings of $3.7 billion.
- Making Medicaid the payer of last resort would produce savings of $31.5 billion.
- Reducing waste, fraud and abuse through greater state vigilance would produce savings of an unknown but substantial amount.

Introduction

Congress cannot balance the federal budget unless the spiraling costs of Medicaid, the nation's health care financing program for the poor, are brought under control. Without fundamental change, over the next seven years the federal government will spend nearly $1 trillion on this one program. Additionally, the states will spend more than $400 million on their share of Medicaid.

The U.S. House of Representatives and the U.S. Senate have agreed on the need to restructure Medicaid, and the key feature of their approach is to provide federal Medicaid funds in block grants to the states. Block-granting Medicaid would allow the federal government to limit the financial exposure of federal taxpayers while, at the same time, giving states maximum flexibility to design a health care program tailored to meet local needs.

Critics have charged that slowing the rate of growth of Medicaid spending, as required by the 1996 Budget Resolution Conference Report,[1] would force states to (1) reduce the number of people covered by Medicaid, (2) reduce the benefits enjoyed by those who continue to be covered, (3) reduce payments to doctors, hospitals and other providers, or (4) some combination of the above. These criticisms are wrong. The purpose of this paper is to show that by adopting sensible reforms Congress can not only meet its budget target but, at the same time, the states can more effectively meet the needs of low-income families.

Medicaid's Financial Crisis

Medicaid is the federal-state health insurance program for the nation's poor. It was created in 1965 as part of the Johnson administration's initiative to expand health insurance to the poor (Medicaid) and elderly (Medicare). Both the federal and state governments provide funds for Medicaid, which is administered by the states under federal guidelines. States match federal funds based on a formula, ranging from as little as 21 cents for each dollar spent in low-income states to 50 cents in high-income states.

Among those entitled to receive Medicaid benefits are recipients of Aid to Families With Dependent Children (AFDC); the aged, blind and disabled receiving Supplemental Security Income (SSI) cash assistance; and pregnant women and children up to age 6 with family incomes less than 133 percent of the poverty level. As a result, the program touches the lives of a great many people:

- Medicaid finances the health care of one out of four American children, and pays for one-third of all U.S. births.
- About 60 percent of those living in poverty are receiving assistance from Medicaid, including 10 percent of the elderly or disabled on Medicare.
- Medicaid pays for about half of all nursing home care.

"Medicaid spending grew at an average annual rate of 19.1 percent between 1990 and 1994."

Medicaid is facing a financial crisis. Even without reform at the federal level, state legislators are already looking for ways to reduce costs. The reason is that Medicaid spending is out of control:

While growth in private-sector health care spending has declined recently, Medicaid spending has continued to explode—growing at an average annual rate of 19.1 percent between 1990 and 1994.[2] [*See Figure I.*]

The Congressional Budget Office (CBO) estimates that federal outlays for Medicaid will be $89.2 billion in 1995, and states will spend an additional $67.3 billion, for a total of $156.5 billion.

Unless Congress reins in the growth of Medicaid, any attempt to balance the federal budget will be futile. The first step in controlling Medicaid spending is to return Medicaid money to the states. The next step is to allow the states to implement some important reforms.

Returning Medicaid to the States

As *Figure II* shows, if the approach proposed by the Republican-led Congress were adopted, the growth in expected Medicaid spending would be significantly lower than has been projected by the CBO and the Office of Management and Budget (OMB). [*See Table I.*] The Clinton administration's recent "balanced budget" also calls for somewhat lower Medicaid outlays.

"By adopting sensible reforms Congress can not only meet its budget target but, at the same time, the states can more effectively meet the needs of low-income families."

Block Grants

As part of Congress' most recent budget plan (the 1996 Budget Resolution Conference Report), Medicaid funds would be given to each state in the form of a block grant:

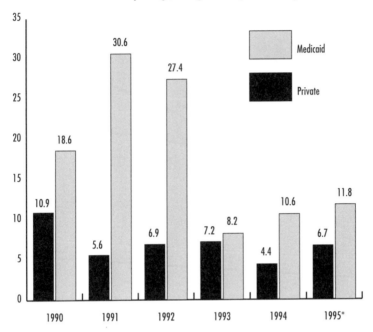

FIGURE I
Health Care Spending (Average annual percent change)

*Projected.
Source: Health Care Financing Administration, Office of the Actuary (includes administrative costs).

TABLE I
Medicaid Outlays, 1995–2002 ($ billions)

	1995	1996	1997	1998	1999	2000	2001	2002
CBO	89.2	99.3	110.0	122.1	134.8	148.1	162.1	177.8
OMB	88.4	95.9	104.6	114.4	124.5	136.5	149.0	163.0
Clinton	88.4	92.0	100.0	109.0	117.0	127.0	138.0	150.0
Congress	89.2	95.7	102.1	106.2	110.5	114.9	119.5	124.3

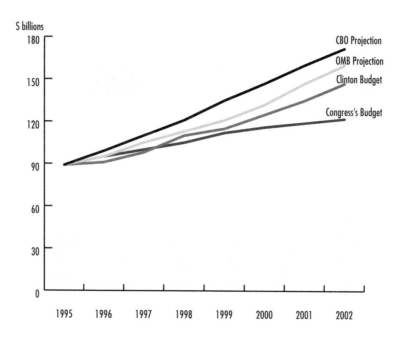

FIGURE II
Medicaid Spending

- Over the seven-year period from 1996 through 2002, total outlays would be $773 billion.[3]
- This would be $329 billion more than the $444 billion spent during the previous seven years (1989–95).[4]
- But it would be $181.6 billion less than the CBO's projection of spending under current law.[5] [See Figure III.]

The Impact of Block Grants
How Medicaid recipients are affected by the block grants will depend upon how the states use the funds. Opponents of reform are predicting dire consequences. According to a recent article in the *Wall Street Journal*:

> [E]xperts on all sides of the issue agree that a 4 percent cap on Medicaid spending won't be enough to cover the expected growth in population in the program. And they say the situation can only result in one or a combination of three things: fewer benefits for Medicaid beneficiaries; lower payments

FIGURE III
Medicaid Spending: The Last Seven Years and the Next ($billions)

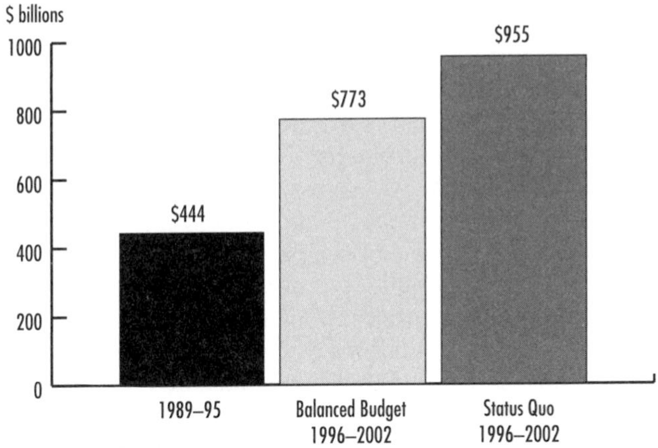

$ billions

Source: Congressional Budget Office.

to doctors, hospitals and other medical care
providers who treat patients in the program; or
reduced eligibility.[6]

*"One of the merits of block grants is that they encourage states to
innovate."*

Such criticisms ignore the fact that one of the merits of
block grants is that they encourage states to innovate and to
improve the way Medicaid operates. In fact, Medicaid savings
can be achieved without reductions in benefits for needy people.
How? By doing the following:

- Change incentives for recipients and providers through
  Medical Savings Accounts and/or managed care.
- Enforce estate recovery provisions.
- Redirect "disproportionate share hospital" payments.
- Reduce administrative costs.
- Make Medicaid the payer of last resort.
- Reduce waste, fraud and abuse through greater state
  vigilance.

Implementing these reforms in the ways explained below would
allow states to provide better health care for the poor—with less
money.

Although only about one-fifth of Medicaid recipients are currently enrolled in a managed care plan, about 93 percent of Medicaid payments are for fee-for-service patients, according to a recent report by Lewin-VHI.[7] As a result, the potential savings from managed care are even greater than the above statistics would suggest. Because most of Medicaid's managed care waivers were granted in the last few years, the programs' costs have not been fully evaluated. An exception is Arizona, which is discussed below. Where evaluations have been completed, ample evidence shows that managed care can reduce Medicaid costs, especially for acute care services physician and hospital visits (both inpatient and outpatient) and prescription drugs."

A General Accounting Office (GAO) report states that "a 1991 analysis of previous evaluations of 25 managed care programs in 17 states concluded that managed care programs . . . were able to achieve modest cost savings." The report also said that for the most reliable evaluations, "approximately 80 percent of the (13) programs reported cost savings ranging from 5 to 15 percent."[8] In addition, the CBO has reported that, for the general population (not just Medicaid), "group/staff HMOs reduce use of medical services by an estimated average of 19.6 percent."[9]

"Managing acute care could save an estimated $37.2 billion over the next seven years."

Some argue that managed care costs are lower only because it is primarily the healthy people who move into managed care, leaving sicker and more expensive patients in the fee-for-service pool. But an analysis of 1992 Health Interview Survey data concluded that "the most striking finding is how little HMOs and indemnity plans differ in the prevalence of chronic conditions."[10]

Case Study: Arizona

Until recently, state efforts to enroll Medicaid recipients in managed care programs have targeted the AFDC population. The Arizona Health Care Cost Containment System (AHCCCS) is an exception in that all recipients are in managed care. Compared with the costs if Arizona were running a typical fee-for-service Medicaid program, the savings are substantial. In the acute care portion of the program, managed care saved about 3.6 percent per year from 1984 through 1988 and 8.3 percent per year from 1989 through 1993.[11]

Potential Savings

As shown in *Table II,* the CBO estimates that over the next seven years (1996 through 2002), spending on Medicaid acute care benefits will total $511.7 billion. Since 93 percent of Medicaid program payments are made on a fee-for-service basis, we can multiply 93 percent of each year's acute care outlays by the savings rate achieved in Arizona to estimate the potential savings to Medicaid. Assuming that the potential savings are achieved from the first year of the Medicaid block grant, our estimate of Medicaid savings for the next seven-year period from managing acute care is $37.2 billion. [See *Table II*.]

Managed care also can yield substantial savings in long-term care. The Arizona Long-Term Care System (ALTCS), begun in December 1988, serves the elderly, the physically and developmentally disabled and the mentally retarded. According to the evaluation report cited above, ALTCS achieved savings of 8 percent in 1990, 15 percent in 1991, 22 percent in 1992 and 21 percent in 1993 over the costs of a traditional Medicaid program. Applying these savings percentages to the long-term care outlays projected by the CBO results in total expected savings of $64 billion from 1996 through 2002. [*See Table III.*]

"Savings from managing long-term care could total $64 billion from 1996 through 2002."

TABLE II
Acute Care Savings Estimate ($ billions)

Year	1996	1997	1998	1999	2000	2001	2002	Total
Acute Care Benefits (CBO)	51.2	57.6	64.7	72.1	80.2	88.6	97.3	511.7
0.93 × Row 1	47.6	53.6	60.2	67.1	74.6	82.4	90.5	457.9
Savings rate*	.036	.083	.083	.083	.083	.083	.083	
Acute care	1.7	4.4	5.0	5.6	6.2	6.8	7.5	37.2

*Based on the savings achieved in Arizona's AHCCCS, 1983–93.

TABLE III
Long-Term Care Savings Estimate ($ billions)

Year	1996	1997	1998	1999	2000	2001	2002	Total
Long-term care (CBO)	35.4	38.8	42.8	47.2	51.7	57.0	62.7	335.6
Savings rate*	.08	.15	.22	.21	.21	.21	.21	
LTC savings	2.8	5.8	9.4	9.9	10.9	12.0	13.2	64.0

*Based on the savings achieved in Arizona's ALTCS, 1990–93.

Summing up:

- The expected savings from managed care are $37.2 billion for acute care plus $64.0 billion for long-term care.
- The total savings would be $101.2 billion over the next seven years.

Medical Savings Accounts

Medical Savings Accounts can create incentives for patients to help control rising Medicaid costs. A typical Medical Savings Account option gives people the opportunity to move from a conventional, low-deductible health insurance plan to one with a high deductible (say $2,000 to $3,000) and to put the premium savings in a personal account. Beneficiaries pay all medical bills up to the deductible from their MSAs and out-of-pocket funds. Catastrophic insurance pays all expenses above the deductible.

Providing MSAs to Medicaid participants would permit beneficiaries to use the funds in their accounts to pay for small and routine health care expenditures, relying on catastrophic health insurance to pay the major bills. Under this approach, Medicaid beneficiaries would control a portion of their own health care dollars and would have incentives to use these dollars wisely.[12]

Recently, legislation introduced in five states (Indiana, Louisiana, Ohio, Oregon and West Virginia), working from a model proposed by the American Legislative Exchange Council, would have provided vouchers to Medicaid recipients. Beneficiaries would have been able to choose among competing health care plans and MSAs would have been one of the options. In addition, Texas has enacted a pilot project to use MSAs for a limited number of Medicaid recipients.[13]

The political difficulty with MSA proposals has been to construct a program in which Medicaid recipients benefit from being prudent health care shoppers, but use remaining funds for constructive purposes. For example, under a 1994 Indiana proposal (which passed in the state's Senate but not the House) Medicaid beneficiaries who incurred less than $3,250 of medical expenses would have been able to use 10 percent of what they did not spend for services such as day care and job training.

Could MSAs for Medicaid recipients save the states money? That is unclear. While there is evidence that adopting MSAs in the private sector has enabled many businesses to reduce their health care costs significantly, there are no operational Medicaid MSAs to be evaluated. However, a new study of Medicare by Mark Litow (Milliman & Robertson) indicates that MSAs combined with managed care can save as much money as managed care alone, or more.[14]

"Medical Savings Accounts combined with managed care can save as much money as managed care alone, or more."

Reform No. 2: Enforce Estate Recovery

Long-term care is one of the fastest-growing segments of the Medicaid budget, increasing about 15 percent per year since 1990. Although the elderly have more assets than any other segment of the population, nearly half of those who enter a nursing home get Medicaid assistance. One reason is that many people either "spend down" or hide their assets in order to qualify for Medicaid's means-tested benefits. The Omnibus Budget Reconciliation Act of 1993 (OBRA) requires each state to look back three years when determining eligibility for long-term care services to see if a Medicaid recipient has transferred money or other assets to other persons, such as their children. Furthermore, when a Medicaid recipient dies, the state is expected to recover some of the past cost of providing long-term care.

"One source has estimated $25 billion in savings over five years if estate recovery provisions were enforced."

Many states have been lax in enforcing these provisions. The result has been that Medicaid-financed nursing home services intended for the elderly poor are sometimes channeled to those with substantial assets. Indeed, books giving instructions on how to qualify for benefits by transferring assets are widely available.[15] Medicaid-covered nursing home services would cost much less if the states enforced the law.[16] Specifically:

- One source has estimated that if the OBRA 1993 provisions were enforced, $25 billion could be saved over five years.[17]
- Extrapolating from that estimate gives a seven-year saving from estate recovery of $35 billion.

Note that the estimated savings from managed care ($101.2 billion) and estate recovery ($35 billion) add up to $136.2 billion. This is equal to about 75 percent of the aggregate reduction in outlays from the CBO baseline needed to meet Congress's budget goal ($181.6 billion).

Reform No. 3: Redirect "Disproportionate Share Hospital" Payments

As noted above, federal spending on Medicaid is growing at an unacceptably high rate. One reason for this rapid growth (totaling 28 percent in 1991 and 29 percent in 1992) was the shifting of states' Medicaid costs to the federal government. According to the *New York Times:*

> The program has become a giant slush fund that governors use to balance budgets or to free up money for other programs. Although Medicaid costs are supposed to be shared, many states have found ways to get more Federal dollars at little or no cost to local taxpayers. One approach used in the past is for a state to enact a new tax on hospitals, add the revenue to its Medicaid budget, demand Federal matching funds and then reimburse the hospitals for the tax by paying them higher Medicaid rates. "We're funding our judicial system, our highway program and everything else out of a Medicaid loophole," said . . . a legislator.[18] Although the Omnibus Budget Reconciliation Acts of 1991 and 1993 restricted such practices, problems persist. Tax loopholes that allow states to manipulate federal matching funds remain.

Another problem involves disproportionate share hospital (DSH) payments. DSH payments refer to a supplemental payment Medicaid makes to hospitals with a disproportionate share of patients who are low-income, either on Medicaid or indigent. Federal DSH payments grew from $547 million in 1990 to $9.9 billion in 1992 and then declined to $8.5 billion in 1995. The CBO estimates that over the next seven years DSH payments will total $70.7 billion. [*See Table IV.*]

"Freezing 'disproportionate share hospital' payments at 1995 levels would save $13.9 billion."

The Senate budget resolution assumes that DSH payments will be frozen at 1995 levels. This assumption allows the Senate to achieve savings of about $13.9 billion over seven years. Even if frozen, DSH payments would still be sufficient to meet legitimate needs, making payments to those hospitals that provide a disproportionate share of care to low-income populations.

TABLE IV
CBO Medicaid Projections ($ billions)

Year	1996	1997	1998	1999	2000	2001	2002	Total
Acute care benefits	51.2	57.6	64.7	72.1	80.2	88.6	97.3	511.7
Long-term care benefits	35.4	38.8	42.8	47.2	51.7	57.0	62.7	335.6
DSH*	8.9	9.4	9.8	10.3	10.5	10.8	11.0	70.7
Administration	3.8	4.2	4.7	5.2	5.7	6.3	6.8	36.7
Total	99.3	110.0	122.1	134.8	148.1	162.6	177.8	954.7

*Disproportionate share hospital (DSH) payments.

Reform No. 4: Reduce Administrative Costs

According to the CBO, Medicaid's 1995 administrative costs will be $3.4 billion. This annual cost will double over the next seven years and reach a seven-year total of $36.7 billion. Administrative savings can be achieved by eliminating requirements that states develop a state plan and receive approval from the Secretary of the Department of Health and Human Services for any changes to the plan. We estimate this change could result in at least a 10 percent savings in administrative costs, amounting to about $3.7 billion.

Reform No. 5: Make Medicaid the Payer of Last Resort

As a public assistance program, Medicaid is intended to pay for health care services only after a Medicaid recipient's private health insurance has been exhausted. Indeed, according to the 1990 Census, more than 13 percent of Medicaid recipients had some health insurance, either an individual policy or coverage provided by an employer. Medicaid also is supposed to pay only after workers' compensation or liability insurers have paid. But state Medicaid programs generally are not recovering such payments from third-party insurers. Finally, noncustodial parents of Medicaid children are to provide health insurance when it is available through their employment. Yet, again states have not vigorously enforced these requirements.

"Recovering payments from third parties could save $31.5 billion."

A series of General Accounting Office (GAO) reports suggests that the amount of funds not being collected by the states is substantial. One recent report estimated that funds owed but not collected were between $500 million and more than $1 billion in 1985.[19] Since total federal Medicaid outlays were $22.7 billion that year, between 2.2 and 4.4 percent of total Medicaid outlays by the states should have been paid by someone else. With total federal Medicaid outlays projected to be $955 billion over the next seven years, a rough estimate of the future savings from this reform would be $21 billion to $42 billion. We will use the midpoint ($31.5 billion) as our seven-year savings estimate.

Reform No. 6: Reduce Waste, Fraud and Abuse

The GAO estimates that the level of waste, fraud and abuse in health care may be as high as 10 percent. Medicaid Fraud Control Units, the FBI and the Health and Human Services Inspector General's office investigate health care fraud, but the investigative resources of all are stretched thin. Further, states may have had a reduced incentive to eliminate waste, fraud and abuse aggressively. The reason is that Medicaid funding is unlimited. Since the states supply as little as 21 cents of each dollar spent, their benefit from eliminating one dollar of waste is as low as 21 cents.

"After block grants, a state will gain a dollar for each dollar of waste eliminated."

By capping the level of federal funding through a block grant, each state's incentive to eliminate waste, fraud and abuse will change. After the block grant, states will gain a dollar for each dollar of waste eliminated. However, reliable estimates of potential savings under this reform are not available.

Conclusion

The six factors discussed above can substantially reduce the cost of Medicaid without adversely affecting Medicaid recipients. As *Table V* shows, the expected total savings over the seven-year period are $185.4 billion.

Block-granting would allow the federal government to limit federal taxpayer exposure for Medicaid costs. This is essential if the federal budget is to be balanced by 2002. Allowing the federal grant to the states to grow at about half of the currently projected rate would provide the states with enough resources to meet the immediate and long-term care needs of the poor, disabled and elderly.

The mechanisms for cost reduction are available now but "absent rigorous federal spending restraints" the states lack

TABLE V
Summary of Savings[a]

Factor	Total
1. System reform:	
Acute care	37.2
Long-term care	64.0
2. Estate recovery	35.0
3. DSH	13.9
4. Administrative costs	3.7
5. Third party collections	31.5
6. Reduce waste, fraud, and abuse	?
Total	185.3

[a]Effects of interaction are not included.

incentives to use them. Federal block grants will provide those incentives.

"Six reforms would meet Congress's budget goals without any reduction in health care benefits for Medicaid beneficiaries."

Notes

1. All references to a particular year of the federal budget refer to the government's fiscal year, which runs from October 1 through September 30.

2. Federal Medicaid outlays grew by 27.8 percent in 1991 and by another 29.1 percent in 1992.

3. The plan assumes Medicaid outlays of $89.2 billion in 1995, with increases held to 7.2 percent in 1996, 6.8 percent in 1997 and 4 percent per year thereafter. The level of proposed spending is compatible with higher growth rates for benefits and administration if disproportionate share hospital payments, which are explained later in this paper, are frozen at 1995 levels.

4. If the block grant spending were compared with Office of Management and Budget (OMB) projections, substantially smaller seven-year Medicaid savings would result from the block grant because the administration assumes slower Medicaid growth. Over the period 1996 through 2002, OMB Medicaid projections are $66.8 billion less (cumulatively) than the CBO projections. Seven-year Medicaid savings from OMB projections would total $114.8 billion under the Budget Resolution Conference Report block-grant assumptions.

5. Based on which projection is used, the block grant proposal promoted by Congress could result in savings of between $114.8 billion and $181.6 billion over the seven-year period between 1996 and 2002.

6. Hilary Stout, "Contrasting Reactions to GOP Proposals to Cut Medicare, Medicaid Reflect Voting Blocs' Power," *Wall Street Journal,* May 30, 1995. The same theme is developed in a Families USA report titled "Hurting Real People: The Human Impact of Medicaid Cuts," Washington, DC, June 1995.

7. Lewin-VHI, "States as Payers: Managed Care for Medicaid Populations," National Institute for Health Care Management, Washington, DC, February 1995.

8. U.S. General Accounting Office, "Medicaid: States Turn to Managed Care to Improve Access and Control Costs," GAO/HRD-93-46, March 1993, p. 39.

9. Based on its analysis of the 1992 National Health Interview Survey, "The Effects of Managed Care and Managed Competition," CBO Staff Memorandum, February 1995, p. 2.

10. Teresa Fama, Peter D. Fox and Leigh Ann White, "Do HMOs Care for the Chronically Ill?" *Health Affairs*, Spring 1995, p. 237.

11. Nelda McCall et al., "Evaluation of Arizona's Health Care Cost Containment System Demonstration," Draft Fourth Outcome Report, submitted to HCFA April 1995.

12. See Brant S. Mittler and Merrill Matthews Jr., "Can Managed Care Solve the Medicaid Crisis?" National Center for Policy Analysis, NCPA Brief Analysis No. 155, April 10, 1995.

13. Molly Hering Bordonaro, "Medical Savings Accounts and the States: Growth From the Grassroots," National Center for Policy Analysis, NCPA Brief Analysis No. 170, August 3, 1995.

14. Mark E. Litow, "Reform Options for Medicare," National Center for Policy Analysis, NCPA Policy Report, forthcoming, August 1995.

15. See, for example, Armond D. Budish, *Avoiding the Medicaid Trap: How to Beat the Catastrophic Cost of Nursing Home Care*, 3rd Ed. (New York: H. Holt, 1995).

16. U.S. General Accounting Office, "Medicaid Estate Planning," GAO/HRD-93-29R, July 20, 1993; and "Medicaid: Recoveries From Nursing Home Residents' Estates Could Offset Program Costs," GAO/HEHS-94-133, August 1, 1994.

17. Marrilyn Serafini, "Plugging a Drain on Medicaid," *National Journal*, March 3, 1995, p. 687.

18. Paul Offner, "Medicaid Games," *New York Times*, May 19, 1995, p. A 31. Also see GAO, "Medicaid: States Use Illusory Approaches to Shift Program Costs to Federal Government," GAO/HEHS-94-133, August 1, 1994.

19. U.S. General Accounting Office, "HCFA Needs Authority to Enforce Third-Party Requirements on States," GAO/HRD-91-60, April 1991. Also see GAO, "Medicaid: Millions of Dollars Not Recovered From Michigan Blue Cross/Blue Shield," GAO/HRD-91-12, November 1990.

Source: National Center for Policy Analysis. http://www.ncpa. org/studies/s197/s197.html. Accessed September 9, 2003.

National Committee for Quality Assurance

http://www.ncqa.org

The NCQA's Web site states that HEDIS® (Health Plan Employer Data and Information Set) is the performance-measurement tool of choice for more than 90 percent of the nation's managed care organizations. It is a set of standardized measures that specify how health plans collect, audit, and report on their performance in important areas ranging from breast cancer screening to helping patients control their cholesterol to customer satisfaction. Although there is a charge for in-depth access to the data, its summary report, The State of Managed Care Quality, 2001, is available via the Web site. Its table of contents is reproduced below.

The State of Managed Care Quality, 2001
Table of Contents

I. *Introduction*
    1. About the State of Managed Care Quality Report
    2. Managed Care and the U.S. Health Care Industry

II. *Key Findings*
    1. About HEDIS®
    2. Patterns of Change Over Time

        i.   Incremental Increases
        ii. Sharp Increases
        iii. Decreasing Variability

    3. Improvement in Heart Disease Measures
    4. Improvement in Women's Health Measures
    5. Improvement in Patients' Experiences with Health Plans

        i.   Consistently High Performance
        ii. Steady Increase
        iii. Substantial Increases

    6. Opportunities for Improvement

III. *Measure-by-Measure Reports*
    1. Adolescent Immunization Status
    2. Advising Smokers to Quit
    3. Use of Appropriate Medication for People with Asthma
    4. Beta Blocker Treatment After a Heart Attack
    5. Breast Cancer Screening
    6. Cervical Cancer Screening
    7. Childhood Immunization Status
    8. Chlamydia Screening in Women

9. Cholesterol Management After Acute Cardiovascular Events
10. Comprehensive Diabetes Care
11. Controlling High Blood Pressure
12. Follow-Up After Hospitalization for Mental Illness
13. Management of Menopause
14. Prenatal and Postpartum Care

IV. *Consumer Experiences in Managed Care Organizations: Results from the 2001 CAHPS® 2.0H Survey*
1. 2001 CAHPS® 2.0H: Purpose and Methodology
2. 2001 CAHPS® 2.0H Composites and Overall Ratings: National Trends and Regional Analyses
3. 2001 CAHPS® 2.0H: Analysis of Individual Items
4. CAHPS® 2.0H Survey Results for Preferred Provider Organizations (PPO)

V. *The Business Case for Quality*
1. Introduction
2. Direct vs. Indirect Costs
3. HEDIS: Measuring What Matters
4. The Quality Dividend Calculator: Using HEDIS and Accreditation to Quantify Savings
5. Case Study: Comprehensive Diabetes Care
6. The Productivity Dividend
7. Bibliography

VI. *Appendix Tables*
1. Comparing the HEDIS 2001 Results of Accredited/ Not Accredited HEDIS Participants
2. Comparing the HEDIS 2001 Results of Public Reporting/Not Public Reporting HEDIS Participants
3. Impact of Rotation on HEDIS 2001 Results

Source: National Committee for Quality Assurance. http://www.ncqa. org/communications/publications/hedispub.htm. Accessed January 27, 2003.

New Democrats Online

http://www.ndol.org/

New Democrats Online (NDOL.org) is the shared online home of the Democratic Leadership Council. Its Health Care page provides position papers on health and health reform–related topics. Often the material included on this Web site is taken from other groups, and this site is often a repository of health policy–related material from a more centrist to liberal perspective interested in expansion of health insurance coverage. The example of its material included here is the report "A Performance-Based Approach to Universal Health Care," which was a proposal prepared for the Covering America project conducted by the Economic and Social Research Institute (ESRI) and funded by The Robert Wood Johnson Foundation. This report focuses on the issue of accountability and how to create a framework for that as part of an approach toward universal health care.

A Performance-Based Approach to Universal Health Care

Policy Report November 15, 2002
By David Kendall, Jeff Lemieux and S. Robert Levine
Editor's Note: This proposal *was one of 13 prepared for the Covering America project, conducted by the Economic and Social Research Institute (ESRI) and funded by The Robert Wood Johnson Foundation. The proposals were published in* Covering America: Real Remedies for the Uninsured, *Volumes 1 and 2. All 13 proposals are available at the ESRI web site at:* www.esresearch. org/covering_america.php.

Overview

For as long as health insurance rates have been measured systematically in the United States, there has been no progress in reducing the number of uninsured. Even after slight improvements in coverage rates at the tail end of arguably the strongest economy in the nation's history, coverage rates are still lower now than they were in 1987. Failure is all too common in health care policy and reform efforts.

Covering the uninsured requires a new approach to health policy. Current policies are based on propagating rules and manipulating behavior, rather than on achieving results. For example, Medicaid provides substantial federal funding in exchange for compliance with federal requirements. Yet, even where federal law requires coverage for certain categories, such as low-income, pregnant women and children, there is no automatic assessment of how effective state efforts are to enroll people. Not surprising, large gaps between eligibility and enrollment rates persist, especially in the case of children.

Rules and incentives are necessary and important tools, but they are more useful in helping to set the conditions for success than as ends in themselves. Health policy needs to include real-time assessment of performance and continuous recalibration of methods to achieve the desired outcome. *Describing success* so everyone can help to pursue it is more likely to inspire progress than merely *prescribing behavior* based on an incomplete theory or an inappropriate model.

Our vision of success is that nearly all U.S. residents have health care coverage, which they select for themselves and which provides them with a level of coverage that is appropriate to their health status and income level. Health care would be delivered safely without waste and with the best possible individual and population-based outcomes. People who remain uninsured for whatever reason would be assured access to community-based outpatient and preventive care services rather than having to rely on emergency room and hospital-based care only, often delivered too late in the course of illness to be effective.

In general, the government would ensure that everyone has the opportunity to get coverage, and individuals would be responsible for obtaining it and using resources wisely. We seek broad recognition that as a community, decisions about the use of health care resources affect our common health and our common wealth.

There can be no real progress or success without clearly defined accountability. Our framework for accountability is straightforward: The federal government provides a basic level of subsidy to everyone according to need and supports the research and encourages the information flow necessary for high-quality, cost-effective use of health care services. The states make sure that coverage is affordable and a choice of health plans is available to people in diverse circumstances. Employers act as conduits for enrolling and paying for coverage (even if they choose to make no contribution themselves), and individuals are responsible for securing coverage and paying their fair share.

Here, then, are the key ingredients of our proposal that are necessary for success:

Tax credits for employer-sponsored and individual health insurance to improve affordability. Our tax credits would apply to both employer-sponsored coverage and individually purchased coverage. They would be available to the uninsured as well as people who are struggling to afford coverage they already have. The existing tax exclusion for employer-sponsored coverage would not be repealed. Therefore, the tax credits would not disrupt employer-sponsored coverage. In addition, the credits would be refundable, which means that low-income workers can use them even if they pay no income tax. They would also be advanceable so workers could use the credit at the time they purchase coverage.

Workplace focus to make coverage easy to get. People are accustomed to getting coverage at work, and our proposal would enable all uninsured workers to do so. However, it would not require employers to sponsor or contribute to coverage.

Voluntary purchasing groups or other options to make choices widely available. As a condition for receiving new federal grants, states would ensure that all employers and individuals could choose among competing group insurance plans through at least one, but preferably several, private purchasing groups. Alternatively, a state could issue a menu of options to make choosing coverage convenient. A modified version of the federal employees' system would be made available to individuals and small businesses as a backup if a state did not follow through.

Performance-based grants to assist states in improving coverage and health care for all their citizens, and to reward those that succeed. All states would receive a base amount to help them improve insurance options in the state, disseminate information about obtaining coverage, advertise the importance of coverage, protect people with high health care costs, and help assure basic care for those who lack coverage. To reward states that succeed, the federal government would give additional grants to states that could document increases in coverage rates. These new state grants would not require state spending to receive federal funding as current programs like Medicaid require. Moreover, these grants would not dictate the means for making improvements. Instead, the federal government would reward states that improve coverage rates so that coverage is equally available and affordable to the young and old, sick and healthy, poor and rich. A portion of the base grant would be set aside for states to participate in national collaborative efforts to develop and test measures of health care quality, access, outcomes, and public health. Those measures would become the basis for additional performance-based grants to states when the data become available.

Information networks to assess state performance, improve quality, and inform policy. In order to fully assess the performance of states, much more data about health care processes and outcomes will be needed. This very same kind of data is important to health professionals, hospitals, and patients in order to avoid costly medical mistakes and to improve quality generally. The same data is also important for research on "the benefit of benefits," which is the subject of controversies involving insurance coverage decisions in the private and public sectors. The federal government would catalyze the creation of information networks that can economically produce this data while keeping patients' medical records private.

Individual responsibility to obtain coverage. With State Children's Health Insurance Program (SCHIP), Medicaid, tax credits, purchasing groups, and the new state grants, coverage for children would be universally available and affordable. A few years after enactment, parents would be denied the personal exemption—a small tax benefit—for any of their children who remained uninsured. As it becomes clear that coverage is more affordable and easy to obtain, adults remaining uninsured would lose their personal exemption as well.

Our plan is divided into two phases to encourage adjustments in federal policy based on a systematic, objective assessment of experience and to allow for an evolution in the political dynamic surrounding issues related to health care coverage. The focus of Phase One is simply getting people coverage through tax credits and performance grants, because some coverage is better than no coverage. Phase One would set in place the accountability framework, rules, and incentives described above. Focusing on the relationship between work and coverage would help correct the misperception that the uninsured are non-workers (most are not). It also would help bind together the interests of the middle class with those who are trying to enter the middle class by making health care coverage more secure for everyone.

The focus of Phase Two is solving the problem of *under*insurance (inadequate benefits for a given health condition or income level) and enforcement of an individual mandate for coverage for all adults—explicitly shifting the burden of responsibility for having coverage to the individual. Five years after our proposed tax credits and other reforms went into effect, we propose a commission to study the impact of the credits and performance grants, to recommend changes if necessary, and, most important, to recommend whether to deny uninsured adults the personal exemption on their taxes. Because any coverage mandate must decide what level of coverage is sufficient, the commission would also need to examine the prevalence of underinsurance. Ultimately, the remaining uninsured must take responsibility for their own health coverage. But before we take that final step, we must make health insurance considerably more affordable and easier to acquire than it is today.

Source: New Democrats Online. http://www.ndol.org/ndol_ci. cfm?contentid=251284&kaid=111&subid=137. Accessed on August 20, 2003.

Physicians for a National Health Program
http://www.pnhp.org/

The Basic Information section of the Physicians for a National Health Program's Web site presents brief reports on key issues relating to the need for a national health system, and its News and Updates section contains press releases and news updates from 1995 to the present. Two of the group's documents are included here. The first is a brief report, "Single-Payer Myths; Single-Payer Facts," that succinctly presents the organization's overall approach to healthcare reform. The second document, "Why the U.S. Needs a Single Payer System," is a more detailed and documented analysis of the advantages this group sees in a single-payer system.

Single-Payer Myths; Single-Payer Facts

Facts about National Health Insurance (NHI) You Might Not Know

The health care delivery system remains private. As opposed to a national health service, where the government employs doctors, in a national health insurance system, the government is billed, but doctors remain in private practice.

A national health insurance program could save approximately $150 billion on paperwork alone. Because of the administrative complexities in our current system, over 25% of every health care dollar goes to marketing, billing, utilization review, and other forms of waste. A single-payer system could reduce administrative costs greatly.

Most businesses would save money. Because a single-payer system is more efficient than our current system, health care costs are less, and therefore, businesses save money. In Canada, the three major auto manufacturers (Ford, GM, and Daimler-Chrysler) have all publicly endorsed Canada's single-payer health system from a business and financial standpoint. In the United States, Ford pays more for its workers health insurance than it does for the steel to make its cars.

Under NHI, your insurance doesn't depend on your job. Whether you're a student, professor, or working part-time raising children, you're provided with care. Not only does this lead to a healthier population, but it's also beneficial from an economic standpoint: workers are less-tied to their employers, and those that dislike their current positions can find new work (where they would be happier and most likely more productive and efficient).

Myths about National Health Insurance (NHI)

The government would dictate how physicians practice medicine. In countries with a national health insurance system, physicians are rarely questioned about their medical practices (and usually only in cases of expected fraud). Compare it to today's system, where doctors routinely have to ask an insurance company permission to perform procedures, prescribe certain medications, or run certain tests to help their patients.

Waits for services would be extremely long. Again, in countries with NHI, urgent care is always provided immediately. Other countries do experience some waits for elective procedures (like cataract removal), but maintaining the US's same level of health expenditures (twice as much as the next-highest country), waits would be much shorter or even non-existent.

People will overutilize the system. Most estimates do indicate that there would be some increased utilization of the system (mostly from the 42 million people that are currently uninsured and therefore not receiving adequate health care), however the staggering savings from a single-payer system would easily compensate for this. (And remember, doctors still control most health care utilization. Patients don't receive prescriptions or tests because they want them; they receive them because their doctors have deemed them appropriate.)

Government programs are wasteful and inefficient. Some are better than others, just as some businesses are better than others. Just to name a few of the most successful and helpful: the National Institutes of Health, the Centers for Disease Control, and Social Security. Even consider Medicare, the government program for the elderly; its overhead is approximately 3%, while in private insurance companies, overhead and profits add up to 15–25%.

Source: Physicians for a National Health Program. http://www.pnhp. org/facts/singlepayer_myths_singlepayer_facts.php. Accessed August 21, 2003.

Why the U.S. Needs a Single Payer Health System

by David U. Himmelstein, MD, and Steffie Woolhandler, MD

Our pluralistic health care system is giving way to a system run by corporate oligopolies. A single payer reform provides the only realistic alternative.

A few giant firms own or control a growing share of medical practice. The winners in the new medical marketplace are determined by financial clout, not medical quality. The result: three or four hospital chains and managed care plans will soon corner the market, leaving physicians and patients with few options. Doctors who don't fit in with corporate needs will be shut out, regardless of patient needs.

A single firm—Columbia/HCA—now owns one quarter of all Florida hospitals, and has announced plans to move into

Massachusetts. In the past year alone the firm has purchased more than a dozen hospitals in Denver and Chicago, closing unprofitable ones and shutting out unprofitable physicians and patients.

In Minnesota, the most mature managed care market, only three or four plans and three or four hospital chains are left. In many rural areas a single plan dominates the market, presenting patients and physicians with a take it or leave-it choice.

Managed care plans in California, Texas and Washington, DC have "delisted" thousands of physicians—both primary care doctors and specialists—based solely on economic criteria. One Texas physician was featured in Aetna's newsletter as "Primary Care Physician of the Month," and thrown out of the plan shortly thereafter when he accumulated high cost patients in his practice. In Massachusetts, BayState HMO "delisted" hundreds of psychiatrists, instructing their patients to call an 800 number to be assigned a new mental health provider. The for-profit firm running Medicaid's managed mental health care plan has just informed psychiatrists that many of them will be barred from the plan as a cost cutting measure.

HMOs are racing to take over Medicare, despite evidence that HMOs have actually increased Medicare costs. The managed care plans sign up mainly the healthy elderly, often illegally inquiring about their health history. The physician contracts offered by plans such as Secure Horizons/Tufts virtually exclude small practices as well as academic physicians who practice less than full time. Financial incentives that penalize the primary care physician for every specialty referral, diagnostic test, and hospital visit pit patients against doctors, and specialists against primary care physicians.

HMOs/insurers that can raise massive amounts of capital by selling stock have a decisive advantage. Their deep pockets allow them to mount massive ad campaigns, market nationally to large employers, and set premiums below costs until competitors are driven out. Once they've cornered the market they can drive hard bargains with hospitals and doctors. As a result not-for-profit plans across the country are going for-profit (even Blue Cross), and small plans are being taken over. Even the largest physician-owned plans cannot compete with U.S. Healthcare, Prudential and similar firms with multibillion dollar war chests.

Large drug firms are preparing to directly take over much of specialty care. Merck, Lilly and others are developing "Disease Management" subsidiaries to sub contract with HMOs to care for patients with expensive chronic diseases such as depression, diabetes, asthma and cancer.

A single payer system would save on bureaucracy and investor profits, making more funds available for care.

Private insurers take, on average, 13% of premium dollars for overhead and profit. Overhead/profits are even higher, about 30%, in big managed care plans like U.S. Healthcare. In contrast, overhead consumes less than 2% of funds in the fee-for-service Medicare program, and less than 1% in Canada's program.

Blue Cross in Massachusetts employs more people to administer coverage for about 2.5 million New Englanders than are employed in all of Canada to administer single payer coverage for 27 million Canadians. In Massachusetts, hospitals spend 25.5% of their revenues on billing and administration. The average Canadian hospital spends less than half as much, because the single payer system obviates the need to determine patient eligibility for services, obtain prior approval, attribute costs and charges to individual patients, and battle with insurers over care and payment.

Physicians in the U.S. face massive bureaucratic costs. The average office-based American doctor employs 1.5 clerical and managerial staff, spends 44% of gross income on overhead, and devotes 134 hours of his/her own time annually to billing. Canadian physicians employ 0.7 clerical/administrative staff, spend 34% of their gross income for overhead, and trivial amounts of time on billing[2] (there's a single half page form for all patients, or a simple electronic system).

According to U.S. Congress' General Accounting Office, administrative savings from a single payer reform would total about 10% of overall health spending. These administrative savings, about $100 billion annually, are enough to cover all of the uninsured, and virtually eliminate co-payments, deductibles and exclusions for those who now have inadequate plans—without any increase in total health spending.

The current market-driven system is increasingly compromising quality and access to care.

The number of uninsured has risen rapidly, to 39.7 million nationally [update: This figure is now over 42 million!]. The proportion of people with coverage paid by an employer is dropping, and those with employer-paid coverage face rising out-of-pocket costs. Only massive Medicaid expansions—$10.5 million nationally since 1989—have averted a much larger increase in the uninsured. Proposals for welfare reform and Medicaid managed care programs would shrink Medicaid enrollment (increasing the number of uninsured) and threaten the quality of care for those left on Medicaid.

U.S. Healthcare and other investor-owned managed care plans are inserting "gag" clauses in physicians' contracts. Our own U.S. Healthcare contracts forbid physicians to "take any action or make any communication which undermines or could undermine the confidence of enrollees, potential enrollees, their employers, their unions, or the public in U.S. Healthcare or the quality of U.S. Healthcare coverage" and forbid any disclosure of the terms of the contract. Meanwhile, Leonard Abramson, U.S. Healthcare's CEO, took home $20 million in a single year, and holds company stock valued at $782 million.

Insurers are gutting mental health benefits, denying needed care, cutting payment rates, and insisting on the cheapest—and often not the best—form of therapy.

HMOs have sought to profit from Medicare and Medicaid contracts by providing substandard care, and even perpetrating massive fraud. The largest Medicare HMO, IMC in Florida, induced thousands of the elderly to sign over their Medicare eligibility and then absconded with $200 million in federal funds. Nationwide, Medicare HMOs provide strikingly substandard homecare and rehabilitation to the disabled elderly. Tennessee Medicaid HMOs have failed to pay doctors and hospitals for care.

After 360,000 women and children were enrolled (and $650 million was spent annually), Florida suspended enrollment in its Medicaid HMO program because of flagrant abuses. Administrative costs consumed more than 50% of Medicaid spending in at least 4 Florida HMOs. In one plan that enrolled 48,000 Medicaid recipients, 19% of total Medicaid dollars went for the three owners' salaries. Thousands of patients were denied vital care; sales reps often illegally pressured healthy people into joining HMOs, while discouraging those who were ill; patient complaints, and inspectors' findings of substandard care were repeatedly ignored. Overall, a cursory state audit found serious problems at 21 of the 29 HMOs participating in the program. A more extensive evaluation is just beginning. These Florida scandals are a virtual replay of California's earlier Medicaid HMO experience.

HMO payment incentives increasingly pressure primary care physicians to avoid specialty consultations and diagnostic tests. In this coercive climate, errors of judgment will inevitably occur, denying patients needed specialty care, while specialists are idle. In some areas of the nation (e.g. New York City and California) market imperatives have led to growing unemployment of physicians, while huge numbers of patients don't get adequate care.

Surveys show that patients greatly prefer care in the small-scale, non-institutional practices that are being wiped out in the current system.

A single payer system is better for patients and better for doctors. Canada spends $1000 less per capita on health care than the U.S., but delivers more care and greater choice for patients. Combining the single payer efficiency of Canada's system with the much higher funding of ours would yield better care than Canada's or ours at present.

Canadian patients have an unrestricted choice of doctors and hospitals, and Canadian doctors have a wider choice of practice options than U.S. physicians.

Canadians get more doctor visits and procedures, more hospital days, and even more bone marrow, liver and lung transplants than Americans.

While there are waits for a handful of expensive procedures, there is little or no wait for most kinds of care in Canada. An oft-cited survey that alleged huge waiting lists counted every patient with a future appointment as "in a queue." (The fringe group that conducted the survey also advocates the abolition of the licensing of physicians to open up free competition among "healers.") More legitimate research shows that the average waiting time for knee replacement in Ontario is 8 weeks, as compared to 3 weeks in the U.S. But patient satisfaction levels with the procedure and care are identical. The time from first suspicion to definitive therapy for breast cancer is actually shorter in British Columbia than in Washington State. There are virtually no waits for emergent coronary artery surgery in Canada, though elective cases face delays, particularly with the surgeons held in highest regard. Interestingly, though Canadian MI patients receive substantially fewer invasive diagnostic and therapeutic procedures, death and reinfarction rates are comparable in the two nations. Finally, under a single payer system we would face much less restraint on care than Canada because we spend (and would certainly continue to spend) much more, and have many more specialists and high tech facilities. Hence even the modest limitations on care seen in Canada are unlikely here.

Surgical outcomes for the elderly (all of whom are insured in the U.S.) are, on average, slightly better in Canada.

Surveys show that Canadian doctors are far happier with their system than we are with ours. According to a 1992 poll, 85% prefer their system to ours; 83% rate the care in Canada as very good or excellent, and most physicians would urge their children to enter the profession. Fewer than 300 out of Canada's 50,000 physicians emigrate to the U.S. each year, and a survey of doctors who have practiced in both nations shows a clear preference for the Canadian system. Medicine has remained an extremely desirable profession; medical school admission is even more competitive in Canada than here.

Surveys show very high patient satisfaction in Canada. 96% prefer their system to ours, and 89% rate care good or excellent (up from 71% 4 years ago).

Canadian physicians' incomes are comparable, in most specialties, to those in the U.S., and have kept pace with inflation for the past 25 years.

It is perhaps comforting to know that Canada's highly regarded and efficiently managed health system is run by a government no more competent nor popular than our own. Their postal service and public railroad system generally receive lower marks than ours; their government's record on fiscal management is not better than ours; and polls show that Canadians distrust their government even more than we do.

Many of us have negative feelings toward government, and examples of government inefficiency and incompetence abound. Yet the record of private insurers is far worse. Their overhead is, on average, 600% above that of public programs, and no private insurer's overhead is as low as Medicare's. Dozens of financial scandals have wracked insurers and HMOs in the past year alone (our personal favorite is the $500,000 travel budget consumed by the head of one Blue Cross plan, including a $7000 junket to Africa to lecture on insurance fraud). Moreover, Medicare treats doctors and patients more respectfully than most private insurers, funds virtually all residency training, and pays Massachusetts hospitals higher rates than do most HMOs.

Finally, when a public program misbehaves we have channels to seek redress; we know where Congress meets, and can vote them out. For-profit firms must answer only to their stockholders.

References

1. U.S. Healthcare 1994 Annual Report.
2. *NEJM* 1991; 324:1253.
3. *NEJM* 1993; 329:400–3.
4. U.S. General Accounting Office. Canadian Health Care: Lessons for the U.S. 1991.
5. Data from U.S. Census Bureau, Current Population Survey March Supplement.
6. U.S. Healthcare primary care physician contract.
7. *Modern Healthcare,* 5/1/95:60.
8. Health Care Financing Review 1994; 16:187.
9. Fort Lauderdale *Sun Sentinel.* Florida's Medicaid HMOs: Profits from Pain. 12/11–12/15, 1994 and State Health Watch April 1995.
10. *JAMA* 1993; 270:835.
11. *NEJM* 1990; 323:884.
12. *NEJM* 1993; 328:772.
13. *NEJM* 1994; 331:1063, *Ann Int Med* 1992; 116:507, and OECD Health Database.
14. *Waiting Your Turn.* Fraser Institute, 1994.
15. *NEJM* 1994; 331:1068.
16. *Medical Care* 1993; 34:264.
17. Health Affairs 1991; 10(3):110.
18. *NEJM* 1993; 328:779.
19. *Health Affairs,* Summer 1992:61.
20. *Toronto Globe and Mail,* 10/23/92.
21. *American J Public Health* 1993; 83:1544.
22. Medical school application statistics from JAMA medical education issue, multiple years.
23. *Toronto Star,* 9/13/93.
24. *NEJM* 1990; 322:562.

Source: Physicians for a National Health Program. http://www. pnhp.org/facts/why_the_us_needs_a_single_payer_health_system.php. Accessed on August 21, 2003.

RAND Corporation

http://rand.org/

The report "Health Care Coverage for the Nation's Uninsured" is a good example of the types of reports produced by the RAND Corporation. This report focuses on how to cover the nation's uninsured and whether, if in doing so, the country would move closer to universal coverage. The report draws upon data collected by other groups, such as The Robert Wood Johnson Foundation, and explores issues of insurance utilization, health status, and demographic information. The report highlights the variation across states in the numbers of uninsured and the corresponding issues of access to care, and concludes that many states may need federal assistance to expand access.

Health Care Coverage for the Nation's Uninsured

Can We Get to Universal Coverage?

The goal of expanding public health insurance programs is to provide coverage to most of the nation's uninsured. But policymakers face a number of challenges in determining whether this goal can be reached. For example, how much will it cost? How should new public programs be financed? How will benefits be distributed? Can expanding insurance be left up to the states?

These and related issues are explored in a series of studies by economists Stephen Long and Susan Marquis. Their work draws on data from the Robert Wood Johnson Foundation (RWJF) Family Health Insurance and Employer surveys, conducted in 1993–1994 in Colorado, Florida, Minnesota, New Mexico, New York, North Dakota, Oklahoma, Oregon, Vermont, and Washington. Collectively, these states are similar to all states in their health care systems and population characteristics, and span the variation observed in all 50 states in important population and health policy characteristics. The surveys, which Long and Marquis designed in collaboration with leading survey organizations, compiled extensive insurance, utilization, health status, and demographic information.

Among key study findings to date:

- States vary substantially in the number of uninsured residents and in their population's health and access to care.
- As a consequence, effects of policies will vary across states.
- Many states may need federal assistance to expand access.

How Much Will It Cost States to
Expand Health Insurance Coverage?

Many states have proposed or implemented programs to provide insurance to low-income, uninsured residents. How much will these programs cost?

Long and Marquis estimated eligibility and costs for three programs illustrative of those enacted or under consideration. The number of people who would be eligible for the new programs ranges from 6 to 10 percent of the 10 RWJF survey states' combined population, depending on the specific program parameters. The cost of the expanded coverage in the 10 states combined ranges from about $4.3 to $7.9 billion, depending on program features. This represents 3 to 5 percent of total personal health care spending in the 10 states.

But aggregate estimates mask substantial variation. Indeed, health problems cluster within states: Residents of states with the highest percentage of uninsured are more likely to be in ill health and to have more severe problems with access to care.

The percentage of the nonelderly population without insurance coverage varies substantially, ranging from 27 percent in New Mexico to 10 percent in Minnesota. However, across all 10 of the RWJF survey states, the percentage of the population with public coverage varies little. Thus, the interstate spread of the noninsured stems from variations in the rate of private coverage.

Long and Marquis took a detailed look at the interactions among insurance coverage, health status, and access to care. They grouped the three states with the highest percentage of uninsured persons (Florida, New Mexico, and Oklahoma) and the three having the lowest (Minnesota, North Dakota, and Vermont). They used these groupings to characterize access and health status in states with similar uninsured rates. The following profiles emerge.

Health status: Persons living in states with a higher percentage of uninsured are about twice as likely to be reported in fair or poor health as those living in states with a lower percentage.

Access to care: Residents in states with a higher percentage of uninsured have less access to care. Figure 1 shows variation in several measures of access separately for children and adults. The first two measures (no usual source of care and no

FIGURE 1
Access to Care Varies Substantially Across States

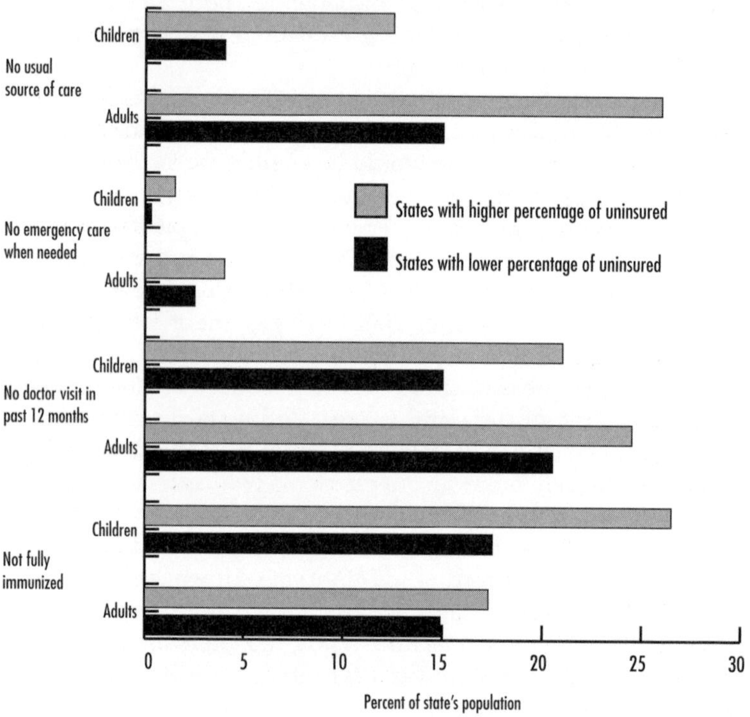

Percent of state's population

Legend:
- States with higher percentage of uninsured
- States with lower percentage of uninsured

emergency care when needed) are about two to three times higher in the high-uninsured states.

Can Federal Policies Help?

Because of differences such as those described above, policies designed to expand health care coverage will have different effects in different states. One example:

Long and Marquis investigated a prototype plan similar to the State Children's Health Insurance Program (CHIP), a federal-state partnership intended to extend health care coverage to a significant proportion of the nation's uninsured children.

Expanding public insurance would substantially improve access for low-income uninsured children. On average, across all 10 RWJF states, a CHIP-like plan would increase physician contact from 2.3 to 4.6 visits per year. But the increase in visit rates for uninsured children would vary significantly, ranging from lows of 41 percent in Minnesota and 50 percent in New York to highs of 135 percent in New Mexico and Vermont and 189 percent in Oregon.

A state's safety net capacity, assessed by measures such as public hospital beds as a percentage of total hospital beds and emergency room visits per low-income person, plays an important role in this variation. Predicted access gains for the three states ranking lowest in safety net capacity are 150 percent, whereas the gains are 80 percent for the three states with the highest capacity.

This analysis suggests that a CHIP-like program is likely to boost the number of low-income children who will be newly insured, substantially increase their access to physician services, and do so across the country. But the magnitude of the effects will vary greatly from one state to another. The biggest potential improvements in access to care are in states that have traditionally provided the scantiest health safety nets.

Can the States Go It Alone?

Can independent actions by states, taken collectively, substantially reduce the nation's uninsured? Probably not. Here's why.

States with a high percentage of uninsured face a significant challenge in expanding health insurance coverage. They will have to spend more per capita than other states to attain equivalent outcomes. But they lack the tax capacity to do so.

Long and Marquis used the additional federal income taxes that a family would pay to finance an illustrative national program of subsidized health insurance for low-income persons as a measure of a state's capacity to finance health reform. They compared this measure of tax capacity with the additional state income taxes the family would be required to pay if each state introduced the same program.

They grouped the 48 states of the continental United States into four groups of 12 states, ordered by the uninsured rate in the state. Figure 2 shows the percentage of uninsured in each group, ranging from 10 to 21 percent. It also shows that the illustrative program Long and Marquis considered would extend coverage to most of the uninsured in all of the states, no matter how many uninsured residents a state had initially.

FIGURE 2
Percent of Population That Is Uninsured, Current and with Illustrative Reform

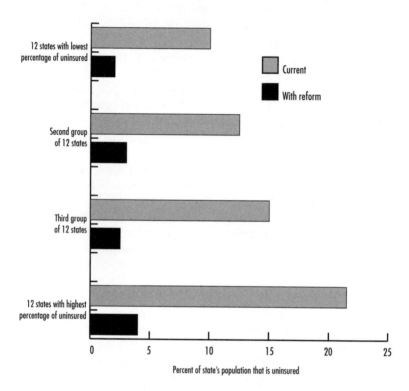

Percent of state's population that is uninsured

How much an extended insurance program will cost is directly related to how many people it will cover; however, the costs can be distributed in different ways. In a national program, they are distributed according to the distribution of family incomes among the states. As a result, per capita taxes are higher in the 12 states with the lowest uninsured rates—about $188— because these states have higher-income populations. In the 12 states with the highest rates of uninsured, the per capita tax increase is about $154; tax increases are lower in these states because they have lower-income populations.

In contrast, under the state-financed plan, costs are distributed according to where the newly insured live. Thus, costs will be higher in states that have more uninsured residents. The estimated per capita tax increase for such states is $230. For residents of the states with the lowest uninsured rates, the average per capita tax increase would be about $130 (in 1993 dollars).

The Long and Marquis analysis illustrates that very unequal programs among the states would result if each state financed a program with a budget limited to its capacity to finance health reform. As Figure 3 shows, the 24 states with the smaller percentage of uninsured would essentially be able to finance the full insurance reform plan because they are also the states with the highest tax capacity. The 24 states with the larger percentage of uninsured would not be able to cover all of their low-income uninsured population with a budget limited to their estimated capacity to finance health system reform.

In sum: the states that most need to expand insurance coverage have the smallest capacity to do so. As a consequence, a strategy relying on incremental, state-by-state action is likely to leave the nation with significant lingering gaps in health care coverage. Some states may need targeted federal assistance—for example, a program like CHIP, which provides federal matching funds to help states implement expanded coverage.

Future Issues

The research by Long and Marquis is helping individual states develop and implement changes in health care financing and delivery that will lead to improved access for the uninsured. But the researchers emphasize that other factors will affect program costs and cost-effectiveness.

For example, on the one hand, not all the people who are eligible enroll in public programs, and participation rates may vary among states because of differences in program implementation. As a result, estimates of program effects may overstate both the number of uninsured who will actually be covered and program costs.

On the other hand, the public program may "crowd out" private insurance. Some families may shift from employer plans to a public program because the latter is cheaper. Or families may lose the opportunity to purchase private insurance—for example, if some employers stop offering insurance because they know that employees can be covered by the public program.

This kind of crowd-out could increase program costs. Moreover, the program would not be reaching the target population—the uninsured.

FIGURE 3
Only Half of the States Can Cover All of Their Uninsured with a
Budget Limited to Their Tax Capacity to Finance Health Reform

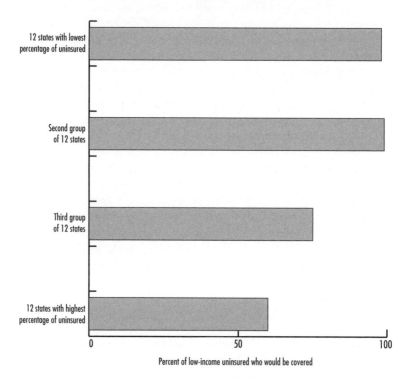

Percent of low-income uninsured who would be covered

Long and Marquis will use data from before and after the expanded programs to cast light on these, and other, critical issues.

For more information:

Cantor, Joel C., Stephen H. Long, and M. Susan Marquis. 1998. "Challenges of State Health Reform: Variations in Ten States." *Health Affairs* 17(1):191–200.

Long, Stephen H., and M. Susan Marquis. 1999. "Geographic Variation in Physician Visits for Uninsured Children: The Role of the Safety Net." *JAMA* 281(21):2035–2040.

Long, Stephen H., and M. Susan Marquis. 1996. "Some Pitfalls in Making Cost Estimates of State Health Insurance Coverage Expansions." *Inquiry* 33(1):85–91.

Marquis, M. Susan, and Stephen H. Long. 1997. "Federalism and Health System Reform: Prospects for State Action." *JAMA* 278(6):514–517.

Selected Bibliography: Increasing Health Care Coverage for the American People

Acs, G., S.H. Long, M.S. Marquis, and P.F. Short. 1996. "Self-Insured Employer Health Plans: Prevalence, Profile, Provisions, and Premiums." *Health Affairs* 15(2):266–278.

Cantor, J.C., S.H. Long, and M. S. Marquis. 1998. "Challenges of State Health Reform: Variations in Ten States." *Health Affairs* 17(1):191–200.

———. 1995. "Private Employment-Based Health Insurance in Ten States." *Health Affairs* 14(2):199–211.

Coburn, A. F., E. H. Kilbreth, S. H. Long, and M. S. Marquis. 1998. "Urban-Rural Differences in Employer-Based Health Insurance Coverage of Workers." *Medical Care Research and Review* 55(4):484–496.

Coburn, A. F., S. H. Long, and M. S. Marquis. 1999. "Effects of Changing Medicaid Fees on Physician Participation and Enrollee Access." *Inquiry* 36(3):265–279.

Goldman, D., J. Buchanan, and E. Keeler. April 2000. "Simulating the Impact of Medical Savings Accounts on Small Business." *Health Services Research* 35.

Goldman, D., A. Leibowitz, J. Buchanan, et al. 1997. "Redistributional Consequences of Community Rating." *Health Services Research* 32(1):71–86. (Also available as RAND Reprint RP-640, 1997.)

Karoly, L.A., and J. A. Rogowski. 1998. "Retiree Health Benefits and Retirement Behavior: Implications for Health Policy." In U.S. Department of Labor, Pension and Welfare Benefits Administration, *Health Benefits and the Workforce*, Volume 2. Washington, D.C.: U.S. Government Printing Office, Chapter Three, pp. 43–71.

Klerman, J. A. 1997. *Health Insurance Among Children of Unemployed Parents.* Santa Monica, Calif.: RAND, MR-883-DOL.

Long, S. H., and M. S. Marquis. 1999a. "Comparing Employee Health Benefits in the Public and Private Sectors, 1997." *Health Affairs* 18(6):183–193.

———. 1998. "Effects of Florida's Medicaid Eligibility Expansion for Pregnant Women." *American Journal of Public Health* 88(3):371–376.

———. 1993. "Gaps in Employer Coverage: Lack of Supply or Lack of Demand?" *Health Affairs* 12(Supplement):282–293; a similar version appears as "Gaps in Employment-Based Health Insurance: Lack of Supply or Lack of Demand?" in U.S. Department of Labor, Pension and Welfare Benefits Administration, *Health Benefits and the Workforce*. Washington, D.C.: U.S. Government Printing Office, 1992, pp. 37–42.

———. 1999b. "Geographic Variation in Physician Visits for Uninsured Children: The Role of the Safety Net." *JAMA* 281(21):2035–2040.

———. 1999c. "Pooled Purchasing: Who Are the Players?" *Health Affairs* 18(4):105–111.

———. 1996. "Some Pitfalls in Making Cost Estimates of State Health Insurance Coverage Expansions." *Inquiry* 33(1):85–91.

———. 1999d. "Stability and Variation in Employment-Based Health Insurance, 1993–1997." *Health Affairs* 18(6):133–139.

———. 1994. "The Uninsured Access Gap and the Cost of Universal Coverage." *Health Affairs* 13(2):211–220.

Long, S. H., M. S. Marquis, and J. Rodgers. 1998. "Do People Shift Their Use of Health Services over Time to Take Advantage of Insurance?" *Journal of Health Economics* 17(1):105–115.

Marquis, M. S., and S. H. Long. 1997. "Federalism and Health System Reform: Prospects for State Action." *JAMA* 278(6):514–517.

———. 1999a. "The Medicaid Eligibility Expansions in Florida: Effects on Financing and the Delivery System for Maternity Care." *Family Planning Perspectives* 31(3):112–121.

———. 1999b. "Recent Trends in Self-Insured Employer Health Plans." *Health Affairs* 18(3):161–166.

———. 1996. "Reconsidering the Effect of Medicaid on Health Care Services Use." *Health Services Research* 30(6):791–808.

———. 1999c. "Trends in Managed Care and Managed Competition, 1993–1997." *Health Affairs* 18(6):75–88.

———. 1994/1995. "The Uninsured Access Gap: Narrowing the Estimates." *Inquiry* 31(4):405–414.

———. 1992. "Uninsured Children and National Health Reform." *JAMA* 268(24):3473–3477.

———. 1995. "Worker Demand for Health Insurance in the Non-Group Market." *Journal of Health Economics* 14(1):47–63.

Pacula, R. L., and R. Sturm. 2000. "Mental Health Parity Legislation: Much Ado About Nothing?" *Health Services Research* 35.

Rogowski, J. A., and L.A. Karoly. 1998. "COBRA Continuation Coverage: Effect on the Health Insurance Status of Early Retirees." In U.S. Department of Labor, Pension and Welfare Benefits Administration, *Health Benefits and the Workforce,* Volume 2. Washington D.C.: U.S. Government Printing Office, Chapter Four, pp. 73–93.

Studdert, D. M. 1999. "Expanded Managed Care Liability: What Impact on Employer Coverage?" *Health Affairs* 18(6):7–27.

Sturm, R. 1997. "How Expensive Is Unlimited Mental Health Care Coverage Under Managed Care?" *JAMA* 278(18):1533–1537.

Sturm, R., W. Goldman, and J. McCulloch. 1998. "Mental Health and Substance Abuse Parity: A Case Study of Ohio's State Employee Program." *The Journal of Mental Health Policy and Economics* 1:129–134.

Sturm, R., and R. L. Pacula. "State Mental Health Parity Laws: Cause or Consequence of Differences in Use?" *Health Affairs* 18(5):182–193.

Sturm, R. and K. B. Wells. April 2000. "Health Insurance May Be Improving—But Not for Individuals with Mental Illness." *Health Services Research* 35.

Sturm R., W. Zhang, and M. Schoenbaum. 1999. "How Expensive Are Unlimited Substance Abuse Benefits Under Managed Care?" *Journal of Behavioral Health Services & Research* 26(2):203–210.

The research summarized in this *Research Highlight* was supported by the Robert Wood Johnson Foundation, Princeton, N.J.

Source: The RAND Corporation. http://www.rand.org/publications/ RB/RB4527/. Accessed August 21, 2003. Copyright @ RAND 2000. Reprinted with permission.

6

Organizations

Professional Societies and Nonprofit Issue and Advocacy Associations

Academy for Health Services Research and Health Policy
1801 K Street NW, Suite 701-L
Washington, DC 20006-1301
(202) 292-6700
http://www.academyhealth.org

This association is made of individuals and organizations involved in health services research. It works to educate the public on the value of health services research in improving the health of the nation. It also works to represent its members in influencing legislative and administrative policies concerning health services research.

Alliance for Health Reform
1444 I Street NW, Suite 910
Washington, DC 20005-6573
(202) 789-2300
http://www.allhealth.org/

The Alliance for Health Reform is a major coalition studying health reform and how to provide health coverage for all Americans at a reasonable cost. Its Web site provides fact sheets (under the link titled Issues) and in-depth analysis (under the Resources link) on topics relating to health reform.

American Hospital Association (AHA)
1 N. Franklin
Chicago, IL 60606-3421
(312) 422-3000
http://www.aha.org

AHA is the leading national organization representing hospitals and other health care provider organizations and institutions. It works to represent these organizations in the national health care policy debate and in legislative and administrative issues relating to its member organizations.

American Medical Association (AMA)
515 N. State Street
Chicago, IL 60610
(312) 464-5000
http://www.ama-assn.org/

The AMA is the oldest and largest association representing physicians in this country. In addition to activities relating to the practice and standards for physician practice, it also works to educate and represent physicians on major national policy issues relating to health care.

American Nurses Association (ANA)
600 Maryland Avenue SW, Suite 100 W. Washington, DC
    20024-2571
(202) 651-7000
http://www.nursingworld.org

ANA, representing over 120,000 registered nurses is the leading professional organization for the nursing profession. In addition to being actively involved in practice and accreditation issues relating to nursing, its political action represents the nursing perspective on health policy related issues.

American Public Health Association (APHA)
800 I Street NW Washington, DC 20001-3710
(202) 777-2742
http://www.apha.org

APHA is made up of over 32,000 health care professional in a wide range of disciplines who work to protect and support the publics health including individuals who do not access to health care, state and local public health and environmental protection departments, community level health issues and communicable diseases.

Center for Health Care Strategies
P.O. Box 3469
Princeton, NJ 08543-3469
(609) 895-8101
http://www.chcs.org

The Center for Health Care Strategies (CHCS) is an affiliate of The Robert Wood Johnson Foundation that "promotes high quality health care services for low-income populations and people with chronic illnesses and disabilities." The center claims to "achieve this objective through awarding grants and providing 'real world' training and technical assistance to state purchasers of publicly financed health care, health plans, and consumer groups." It directs four national initiatives of The Robert Wood Johnson Foundation: Medicaid Managed Care, State Action for Oral Health Access, Covering Kids and Families: Access Initiative, and Improving Asthma Care for Children. Its publications page contains access to pdf versions of its reports relating to these initiatives.

Center for Studying Health System Change
600 Maryland Avenue, SW, Suite 550
Washington, DC 20024
(202) 484-5261
http://www.hschange.org/

The Center for Studying Health System Change (HSC) is a nonpartisan policy research organization located in Washington, D.C. Its Web site states that the "HSC designs and conducts studies focused on the U.S. health care system to inform the thinking and decisions of policy makers in government and private industry." The site includes an array of statistics and provides access to numerous issue briefs and tracking reports that present information over time on insurance coverage and costs, access to care and local markets, and managed care.

The Commonwealth Fund
One East 75th Street
New York, NY 10021

(212) 606-3800
http://www.cmwf.org

The Commonwealth Fund describes itself as "a private foundation that supports independent research on health and social issues and makes grants to improve health care practice and policy.
The Fund is dedicated to helping people become more informed
about their health care, and improving care for vulnerable populations such as children, elderly people, low-income families, minority Americans, and the uninsured." The Web site provides the
fund's numerous reports in pdf format at no charge.

Employee Benefit Research Institute
2121 K Street, NW, Suite 600
Washington, DC 20037-1896
(202) 659-0670
http://www.ebri.org

The Employee Benefit Research Institute (EBRI) describes itself as
"the only nonprofit, nonpartisan organization committed exclu-
sively to data dissemination, policy research, and education on
economic security and employee benefits."

Families USA
1344 G Street, NW
Washington, DC 20005
(202) 628-3030
http://www.familiesusa.org/site/PageServer

Families USA describes itself as "a national nonprofit, nonpartisan organization dedicated to the achievement of high-quality, affordable health and long-term care for all Americans. Working at
the national, state and community levels," the organization
claims it has "earned a national reputation as an effective voice
for health care consumers for over 15 years." The organization's
Web site contains links to reports and fact sheets on many current
health access and insurance issues.

**George Washington University Center for Health
     Services Research and Policy**
2021 K Street NW, Suite 800
Washington, DC 20006
(202) 296-6922
http://www.gwhealthpolicy.org/chsrp

The George Washington University Center for Health Services Research and Policy describes itself on its Web site as being "dedicated to providing policymakers, public health officials, health care administrators, and advocates with the information and ideas they need to improve access to quality, affordable health care."

Henry J. Kaiser Family Foundation
2400 Sand Hill Road
Menlo Park, CA 94025
(650) 854-9400
http://www.kff.org/

The Henry J. Kaiser Family Foundation is a California-based foundation that is a nonprofit, independent national healthcare philanthropy that focuses on a variety of healthcare and health policy concerns. This group sometimes provides grants to universities and researchers to study important health policy issues.

Heritage Foundation
214 Massachusetts Avenue, NE
Washington, DC 20002-4999
(202) 546-4400
http://www.heritage.org/Research/HealthCare/index.cfm

Founded in 1973, the Heritage Foundation is a research and educational institute—a think tank—whose mission is to formulate and promote conservative public policies based on the principles of free enterprise, limited government, individual freedom, traditional American values, and a strong national defense.

Institute for Health Freedom
1825 I Street, NW, Suite 400
Washington, DC 20006
(202) 429-6610
http://www.forhealthfreedom.org/index.html

The Institute for Health Freedom is a Washington-based think tank looking at the healthcare policy debate from the perspective of maximizing personal freedom in choice of healthcare and in privacy of personal health information.

Institute for Health Policy Solutions
1444 I Street, NW, Suite 900
Washington, DC 20005
(202) 789-1491
http://www.ihps.org

The Institute for Health Policy Solutions describes itself on its Web site as "an independent not-for-profit organization established in April 1992 to identify, analyze, and develop strategies to solve health care system problems. In general, the Institute's work addresses reforms to improve access, contain costs and promote cost-effective financing and delivery systems. Although committed to no ideological perspective, the Institute brings special expertise and interest to approaches that reflect complementary roles for the public and private sectors." The institute's data and reports focus on insurance coverage of children and working families.

Institute of Medicine (IOM)
500 Fifth Street NW
Washington, DC 20001
(202) 334-2352
http://www.iom.edu

The IOM is a nonprofit organization affiliated with the National Academy of Sciences. It is designed to serve as an adviser to the nation to improve health. The Institute provides unbiased, evidence-based, and authoritative information and advice concerning health and science policy to policy-makers, professionals, leaders in every sector of society, and the public at large. It has produced a number of influential reports relating to many aspects of health care organization and delivery. Membership is considered an honor and includes many of the leading policy, research and clinical practice professional in the United States.

National Academy for State Health Policy
50 Monument Square, Suite 502
Portland, ME 04101
(207) 874-6524
http://www.nashp.org

The National Academy for State Health Policy is a nonprofit, nonpartisan organization set up to analyze health reform and policy on the state level.

National Association of Public Hospitals and Health Systems
1301 Pennsylvania Avenue, NW, Suite 950
Washington, DC 20004
(202) 585-0100

The National Association of Public Hospitals and Health Systems represents over 100 hospitals and health systems that together comprise the essential infrastructure of many of America's largest metropolitan health systems. Since its inception in 1980, the NAPH has cultivated a strong presence on Capitol Hill, with the executive branch, and in many state capitols. The association has made significant strides in its twenty-year history in educating federal, state, and local decision makers about the unique needs of and challenges faced by member hospitals and the nation's most vulnerable populations.

National Center for Policy Analysis
601 Pennsylvania Avenue NW, Suite 900, South Building
Washington, DC 20004
(202) 628-6671
http://www.ncpa.org/

The National Center for Policy Analysis is a private policy-oriented group that publishes material on a variety of policy topics, including healthcare policy. The center has a more conservative point of view and lists its mission as "developing and providing private alternatives to government regulation" in a variety of public-policy areas including health, Social Security, welfare, criminal justice, environmental, and educational issues.

National Coalition on Healthcare
1200 G Street, NW, Suite 750
Washington, DC 20005
(202) 638-7151
http://www.nchc.org/

The National Coalition on Healthcare is a nonprofit and self-proclaimed rigorously nonpartisan coalition of almost 96 groups, employing or representing approximately 100 million Americans. Its focus is examining health-related issues to look at ways to achieve better, more-affordable healthcare for all Americans.

National Committee for Quality Assurance
2000 L Street, NW, Suite 500

Washington, DC 20036
http://www.ncqa.org

The National Committee for Quality Assurance (NCQA) provides information about the quality of the nation's managed care plans. It accredits many of the nation's healthcare plans and produces data and reports on the quality of these plans via its HEDIS®—Health Plan Employer Data and Information Set.

National Health Policy Forum
2131 K Street, NW, Suite 500
Washington, DC 20037
(202) 872-1390
http://www.nhpf.org

The National Health Policy Forum (NHPF), located at George Washington University in Washington, D.C., provides a forum for a nonpartisan exchange of ideas between senior government staff and experts from many healthcare settings.

Physicians for a National Health Program
29 East Madison, Suite 602
Chicago, IL 60602
(312) 782-6006
http://www.pnhp.org/

Physicians for a National Health Program is an association of physicians who advocate a single-payer national healthcare system. This group does both issue analysis and advocacy and provides a liberal analysis of how to deal with healthcare reform, given its advocacy of a single-payer system.

RAND Corporation
1700 Main Street
P.O. Box 2138
Santa Monica, CA 90407-2138
(310) 393-0411
http://rand.org/

The RAND Corporation is a major public-policy-oriented research institute that began during World War II and since then has become an independent, nonprofit research and policy organization. The RAND Corporation conducts research on a wide variety of public-policy topics, including healthcare, education, and welfare. Often its reports are results of funded studies by researchers connected with RAND.

UCLA Center for Health Policy Research
10911 Weyburn Avenue, Suite 300
Los Angeles, CA 90024
(310) 794-0909
http://www.healthpolicy.ucla.edu/

The UCLA Center for Health Policy Research is a research center at the University of California, Los Angeles (UCLA), that focuses on the health needs of communities and populations that are at risk for adverse health conditions or are underserved by the health system.

Government Agencies

Agency for Healthcare Research and Policy
540 Gaither Road
Rockville, MD 20850
(301) 427-1364
http://www.ahcpr.gov/

In examining what works and does not work in healthcare, AHRQ's mission includes both translating research findings into better patient care and providing policymakers and other healthcare leaders with information needed to make critical healthcare decisions.

Centers for Disease Control and Prevention
1600 Clifton Road
Atlanta, GA 30333
(404) 639-3534
http://www.cdc.gov/

The Centers for Disease Control and Prevention (CDC) is recognized as the lead federal agency for protecting the health and safety of people at home and abroad, providing credible information to enhance health decisions, and promoting health through strong partnerships. CDC serves as the national focus for developing and applying disease prevention and control, environmental health, and health promotion and education activities designed to improve the health of the people of the United States.

Centers for Medicare and Medicaid Services
7500 Security Boulevard
Baltimore, MD 21244-1850
(877) 267-2323
http://www.cms.hhs.gov/

CMS is the federal agency responsible for administering the Medicare, Medicaid, SCHIP (State Children's Health Insurance), HIPAA (Health Insurance Portability and Accountability Act), CLIA (Clinical Laboratory Improvement Amendments), and several other health-related programs.

Health Resources and Services Administration
U.S. Department of Health and Human Services
Parklawn Building
5600 Fishers Lane
Rockville, MD 20857

The Health Resources and Services Administration's mission is to improve and expand access to quality healthcare for all. It is moving toward 100 percent access to health care and 0 health disparities for all Americans. The HRSA seeks to assure the availability of quality healthcare to low-income, uninsured, isolated, vulnerable- and special needs populations and meets their unique healthcare needs. The administration strives to eliminate barriers to care, eliminate health disparities, assure quality of care, and improve public health and healthcare systems.

Indian Health Service
The Reyes Building
801 Thompson Avenue, Suite 400
Rockville, MD 20852-1627
(301) 443-1083
http://www.ihs.gov/

The Indian Health Service's mission is to raise the physical, mental, social, and spiritual health of American Indians and Alaska Natives to the highest level. The service strives to assure that comprehensive, culturally acceptable personal and public health services are available and accessible to American Indian and Alaska Native people. It upholds the federal government's obligation to promote healthy American Indian and Alaska Native people, communities, and cultures and to honor and protect the inherent sovereign rights of tribes.

National Institutes of Health
9000 Rockville Pike
Bethesda, MD 20892
http://www.nih.gov/

Begun as a one-room Laboratory of Hygiene in 1887, the National Institutes of Health (NIH) today is one of the world's foremost medical research centers. An agency of the Department of Health and Human Services, the NIH is the federal focal point for health research. It is the steward of medical and behavioral research for the nation. Its mission is science in pursuit of fundamental knowledge about the nature and behavior of living systems and the application of that knowledge to extend healthy life and reduce the burdens of illness and disability. The goals of the agency are as follows: (1) foster fundamental creative discoveries, innovative research strategies, and their applications as a basis to advance significantly the nation's capacity to protect and improve health; (2) develop, maintain, and renew scientific human and physical resources that will assure the nation's capability to prevent disease; (3) expand the knowledge base in medical and associated sciences in order to enhance the nation's economic well-being and ensure a continued high return on the public investment in research; and (4) exemplify and promote the highest level of scientific integrity, public accountability, and social responsibility in the conduct of science.

Substance Abuse and Mental Health Services Administration
Rm 12-105, Parklawn Building
5600 Fishers Lane
Rockville, MD 20857
(301) 443-4795
http://www.samhsa.gov/

SAMHSA is the federal agency charged with improving the quality and availability of prevention, treatment, and rehabilitative services in order to reduce illness, death, disability, and cost to society resulting from substance abuse and mental illnesses.

7

Selected Print and Nonprint Resources

With the emergence of the Internet and the World Wide Web, public and school libraries are able to make available a much stronger selection of research resources. Additionally, a myriad of research and policy organizations now have their own Web sites, many of which present their own research documents or links to research conducted by others. This chapter will present information on some of these Web and print-based resources. Although your library may not have all of these resources, they should have some of them, as well as additional resources not listed here. When you go to your library, go to the reference desk and ask for assistance in locating information on your topic. Many of these resources are available to you via the Web so that you can access them from home or from wherever you are doing your research.

Books and Government Reports

Although the Internet and the World Wide Web are becoming increasingly important sources for information on many topics, including health reform, books and reports are still important sources of information. They can often give a more in-depth overview and analysis of the topic than can easily be found on the Web. The materials listed below are good sources of information on health reform and are representative of print resources available at this time. When checking with your local library to

233

obtain these resources, be sure to look for other relevant resources available.

Budrys, Grace. 2001. *Our Unsystematic Healthcare System.* Lanham, MD: Rowman and Littlefield Publishers.

This book reviews different topics relating to the U.S. healthcare system for nonacademics. Among the chapters included are: Two Sociological Perspectives of the Healthcare System; Hospitals and Other Healthcare Organizations; Alternative Medicine; Health Insurance; HMOs and Managed Care; Reform; and Healthcare Systems in Other Countries.

Budrys, Grace. 2003. *Unequal Health: How Inequality Contributes to Health or Illness.* Lanham, MD: Rowman and Littlefield.

This book focuses upon the issue of health disparities among Americans. The book contrasts popular beliefs about the importance of factors such as race, poverty, and sex and health habits with academic research on the same topics. In addition, the book explores such topics as access to medical care, genetics, and stress. Several chapters also deal with the relationship between social inequality and health status. The author challenges some of the basic tenets of the American belief system and the ideal that most Americans could improve their health significantly if they chose to do so. Instead, the book shows how health and well-being in American society today are linked to economic status.

Gordon, Colin. 2003. *Dead on Arrival: The Politics of Health Care in Twentieth Century America.* Princeton, NJ: Princeton University Press.

From a historical perspective, this book tries to answer the question of why, alone among its democratic capitalist peers, the United States does not have national health insurance. The book presents three different types of explanations: the liberal or pluralist view, the institutionalist view, and the radical view. The author focuses on the privileged status enjoyed by economic interests in American politics as the major answer, but uses detailed information from past debates and fights to have certain pieces of health-related legislation passed to help answer this question. The book provides details about both the political and ideological clout of leading health interests and the organizational struggles of health reformers.

Health Insurance Association of America. 2002. *Source Book of Health Insurance Data, 2002.* Washington, DC: Health Insurance Association of America.

This book provides data and tables on a range of topics relating to health insurance such as the private health insurance industry; public health coverage; medical care costs; health services, resources, and utilization; and disability, morbidity, and mortality.

Himelfarb, Richard. 1995. *Catastrophic Politics: The Rise and Fall of the Medicare Catastrophic Coverage Act of 1988.* University Park: Pennsylvania State University Press.

This book explores in depth why this legislation ended up being repealed. Upon its enactment in July 1988, the Medicare Catastrophic Coverage Act (MCCA) was initially hailed as the first major expansion of Medicare since its creation in 1965. Only eighteen months later, the House and the Senate, responding to a huge amount of criticism about the legislation, repealed the legislation despite its having been initially supported by President Reagan and the nation's largest senior citizen interest group, the American Association of Retired Persons (AARP). A variety of source materials including interviews with policy makers and surveys of senior citizen opinion are used to help explain why this legislation was repealed.

Institute of Medicine. 2000. *To Err Is Human: Building a Safer Health System.* Washington, DC: National Academy Press.

This book presents a state-of-the-art review of issues in improving the quality of patient care and patient safety. What is meant by errors in healthcare is reviewed, as are the major causes of death and injury and an analysis of why errors occur. The book also discusses error-reporting systems, setting performance standards, and ways to create safer systems in healthcare organizations.

Institute of Medicine. 2001–2003. *Consequences of Uninsurance.* Washington, DC: National Academy Press.

With support from the Robert Wood Johnson Foundation, the Institute of Medicine is completing a three-year, comprehensive study of uninsurance and its implications for uninsured individuals. This project has published six reports from 2001 to 2004 which deal with key issues on the topic. The reports are:

Insuring America's Health: Principles and Recommendations. January 14, 2004
Hidden Costs, Value Lost: Uninsurance in America. June 17, 2003
A Shared Destiny: Community Effects of Uninsurance. March 6, 2003
Health Insurance Is a Family Matter. September 18, 2002
Care without Coverage: Too Little, Too Late. May 21, 2002
Coverage Matters: Insurance and Health Care. October 11, 2001

Johnson, H., and D. S. Broder. 1996. *The System: The American Way of Politics at the Breaking Point.* Boston: Little, Brown.

This book presents a review of the events leading up to the defeat of the Clinton Health Security bill. The book is written by well-known journalists and relies heavily on interviews with many of the people involved in the efforts, including congressional staffers and some elected officials, presidential staff, and staff of the special committees formed by President Clinton to plan the healthcare reform efforts. In addition, the book relies on newspaper and other media coverage of the events. This book focuses upon the internal political aspects of the failure as well as the lack of proper management of support within Congress.

Kronenfeld, Jennie Jacobs. 2002. *Healthcare Policy: Issues and Trends.* Westport, CT: Praeger.

This book, written by one of the authors of the book you are reading, provides an overview and analysis of current key issues in U.S. healthcare policy. Chapters include Physical Health and Disease Trends; Mental Health Concerns and Behavioral Health; The Reorganized U.S. Healthcare System; Healthcare Personnel; Health of Children, Youth and Elderly; Reproductive Health and Abortions; Costs; and Health Reform.

Light, Paul. 1985. *Artful Work: The Politics of Social Security Reform.* New York: Random House.

The book provides a detailed overview of many aspects of the Social Security system from a political perspective. From an interest in health reform, one important portion of the book examines the 1983 Social Security rescue and discusses the lessons from that for the Social Security budget for the future and for the Medicare budget for the future. The review of these past efforts to solidify the financial basis of the program is germane to many of the current debates about the role of Medicare in any type of healthcare reform and about the past ways in which major programs such as Social Security and Medicare have been funded in the United States.

National Organizations of the United States. 2003. *Encyclopedia of Associations.* 39th ed. Farmington, MI: Gale Group.

This resource is available in both print and electronic formats. The database covers national, international, regional, state, and local organizations and contains information on over 135,000 not-for-profit membership organizations. The online database contains all the records, while there are separate print publications for the national; international; and regional, state, and local organizations. The print version will be found in the reference section of most libraries, and the electronic version will be available at selected libraries. The online encyclopedia provides keyword and subject access, while the print version organizes the information alphabetically within each topic.

Navarro, Vincente. 1994. *The Politics of Health Policy: The US Reforms, 1980–1994.* Cambridge, MA: Blackwell Publishers.

This book analyzes the socioeconomic and political forces that explain the federal health policies of the United States in this time period, from a more left-oriented political perspective. The book challenges some of the major positions held in many of the social and political sciences in the United States about the nature of political power in Western capitalist countries and its impact on public policy. The book emphasizes the connection between what Navarro calls "the crisis of health care"—high costs and lack of or limited healthcare coverage—and the correlation of class forces in the United States. In addition, there is discussion of the proposed but not enacted Clinton healthcare reforms from the author's perspective.

Oberlander, Jonathan. 2003. *The Political Life of Medicare.* Chicago: University of Chicago Press.

This book focuses on political developments in Medicare from 1965 to 2002. The focus is on the dynamics surrounding program financing and benefits, in contrast to a number of other studies that have focused on the politics of cost control. The author argues that a variety of tensions have been important in the history of the program. These include a gap between the promise of Medicare as understood by the public (that it should protect the elderly against the potentially devastating costs of medical care) and the actual performance of the program. Other tensions relate to how to find the financing to pay for the costs of the program and the limitations linked to the social insurance financing approach that was adopted to secure Medicare's political success but that has proven to be ill suited, in the author's judgment, to a health insurance program.

Shi, Leiyu, and Douglas A. Singh. 1998. *Delivering Healthcare in America: A Systems Approach.* Gaithersburg, MD: Aspen Publishers.

This book provides an overview of the U.S. healthcare system and its components. Chapters include Beliefs, Values and Health; Health Services Professionals; Medical Technology; Outpatient and Inpatient Facilities and Services; Cost, Access and Quality; and Health Policy.

Skocpol, Thesa. 1997. *Boomerang: Healthcare Reform and the Turn against Government.* New York: W.W. Norton.

This book presents an appraisal by a social scientist of the defeat of the Clinton Health Security bill. In contrast to some other books that focus on the interpersonal and political maneuvers and rely partially on extensive retrospective interviews (see Johnson and Broder 1996), this book began as a paper at a scholarly conference and an article in a scholarly journal. In its shorter form, the article presented the story of the failed effort to pass healthcare reform from the perspective of past and future U.S. domestic politics. The expanded version in the book argues that the health reform bill became an ideal foil for concerted antigovernment countermobilization, led by ideologically committed conservatives.

Williams, Stephen J., and Paul R. Torrens, eds. 2002. *Introduction to Health Services.* 6th ed. Albany, NY: Delmar Publishers.

This book presents seventeen different chapters by leading scholars in the field of health services administration and health services research. Each chapter reads well as stand-alone material. Topics covered include historical evolution and overview of health services in the United States, disease and care-seeking trends, patterns of diseases in the United States, access to care, financing of care, managed care, private health insurance, evolution of public health, ambulatory healthcare services, hospitals, long-term care, mental health services, pharmaceuticals, healthcare professionals, health policy, quality of care, and ethical issues.

Electronic Library-Based Resources

The following resources are electronic products with extensive full-text content that can be accessed by subject. Many public and school libraries make these resources available to their patrons via their library card number. These can be accessed via the Internet from any location. Check your local library to see which are available to you via its system.

EBSCO MasterFILE Premier is designed specifically for public libraries. It provides full text for nearly 1,950 general periodicals covering a broad range of disciplines, including general reference, business, education, health, general science, multicultural issues, and much more. In addition to the full text, this database provides indexing and abstracts for all of the 2,540 publications in the collection. You may search the database by keyword or by subject heading. Under the Healthcare Reform heading, there are 132 newspaper references, 1,723 periodical references, and 8 review references. These are further broken down into over 80 subheadings by subtopic.

Health and Wellness Resource Center is another online resource to full-text information from a variety of resources, including journals, pamphlets, and medical encyclopedias. The Healthcare Reform subject heading has over 3,600 articles and is subdivided into more than 15 subject and geographic headings. In addition, the following health reform topics are covered: cost shifting (medical care); healthcare industry; healthcare rationing; health insurance; health insurance industry; health planning; health policy; and health services administration.

MedlinePlus (http://www.MedlinePlus.gov) is the most important government-sponsored consumer health site. Although available at no charge, many library Web sites provide a link to it, so it is included here. The site is maintained by the National Library of Medicine, the world's largest and most important medical library. In addition to extensive information on specific disease and health conditions, it contains extensive sections relating to health policy issues, including Health Insurance, Medicare, Patient Issues, Mental Health, and Health Professions. The site contains extensive links to National Institutes of Health (NIH) Web sites as well as other quality sites.

NewsBank NewsFile (1991–current) is a full-text database of news articles covering social, economic, environmental, government, sports, health, and science issues and events from more than 500 U.S. regional and national newspapers, wire services, and broadcasts. In addition to being searchable by keyword, there are the following relevant subject headings: Health Insurance, Health Care Reform, Health Care Provision, Health Care Industry, Quality of Care, Nursing Homes, Medical Test Laboratories, Managed Care, Hospice Care, Home Health Care Services, Health Maintenance Organizations (HMOs), Health, Clinics, Medical Records, Medical Personnel, Prenatal Care, Health Insurance Industry, Elder Care, and Dental Care Services. This an excellent source to confirm dates as well as to obtain short discussions of relevant topics.

ProQuest ABI/INFORM is an online business database with extensive full-text entries. The database contains content from thousands of journals that help researchers track business conditions, trends, management techniques, corporate strategies, and industry-specific topics worldwide. ABI/INFORM indexers have an extensive list of more than 8,000 subject headings to use in indexing the articles so that very specific searches can be performed. The most relevant of these subject headings for a general search on health reform is "national health insurance." As is indicated by its business focus, this database provides information on various aspects of health reform from a business perspective.

ProQuest News & Magazines is a digital database offering indexed full-text content from popular magazines and journals, and national and local newspapers. Complete articles are always available in one or more formats. Newspapers and magazines are a good source to find information about events when they happened.

SIRS Publishing inc is a company that provides in both print and electronic formats articles on issues of current interest.

Its articles are selected to provide a balanced view of the topic and for the conciseness, accuracy, and relevance of their content. The content is aimed at a high-school-level audience. The company markets several online products, including the following (this product description is taken from Web site at http://www.sirs.com/products/index.htm):

> SIRS Knowledge Source® (SKS) is a comprehensive database portal which is comprised of several distinct reference databases including SIRS Researcher®, SIRS Government Reporter®, SIRS Renaissance® and SKS WebSelect™ with available links to SIRS Interactive Citizenship™, SIRS Discoverer® and coming soon Discoverer's WebFind™. Updated daily, SKS provides relevant, credible information on social issues, science, history, government, the arts and humanities. Full-text articles and Internet resources are carefully selected from thousands of domestic and international publications and respected organizations.
>
> In SIRS Knowledge Source, the most relevant topic for health reform is in the Domestic Affairs: Health Care Industry section with subtopics of Economics, Ethics, Facilities, Fraud, Insurance, Reform, and Workers. Under the Reform subheading are the subtopics of Health Security, Legislation, Prescription Drugs/Pharmaceuticals, and State/Regional Perspective.

Health Research and Healthcare Policy Organization Web Sites

As indicated in Chapter 5, the following are relevant organizations and issue-oriented Web sites, similar to those presented above. However, due to space limitations sample documents from the following were not included.

AcademyHealth
http://www.academyhealth.org

The AcademyHealth Web site states that it "is the professional home for health services researchers, policy analysts, and practitioners, and a leading, non-partisan resource for the best in health research and policy." The site contains pdf versions of Academy-Health-produced reports on quality issues in healthcare, insurance coverage and strategies, state responses to coverage, and purchasing issues, as well as a good glossary of health service and health reform terms.

Employee Benefit Research Institute
http://www.ebri.org

In the Program section of the Employee Benefit Research Institute's Web site, three sections relevant to health appear: Consumer Health Education Council, which includes a section with information on the uninsured; Health Confidence Survey, with results back to 1997; and The Health Security and Quality Research Program, which produces print reports used in health policy analysis.

George Washington University Center for Health Services Research and Policy
http://www.gwhealthpolicy.org/chsrp

This site provides free, electronic access to a large number of reports it produces as well as access to reports produced by other groups. Typical focuses of the reports include federal and state legislation, laws, and policies; managed care contracting; Medicaid, CHIP, and Medicare; HIV/AIDS; safety net provider and underserved populations; welfare reform; people with disabilities; and maternal and child health.

Institute for Health Freedom
http://www.forhealthfreedom.org/index.html

Its Web site provides access to press releases and reports on the different aspects of healthcare from the organization's perspective.

Moving Ideas Network
http://www.movingideas.org

Moving Ideas Network (MIN), formerly the Electronic Policy Network!, is an organization that tries to bring to a wider audience the resources and work of progressive research and advocacy organizations. Under the Weekly Round Up section of the Web page are links to reports by subject. Under Healthcare Policy, there are annotated links to over 200 full-text reports on health policy and reform issues from a conservative perspective.

National Academy for State Health Policy
http://www.nashp.org

The academy's Web site makes available in pdf format a range of reports that it has produced on the various health policy–related issues and how states should deal with them.

National Association of Public Hospitals and Health Systems
Issues Advocacy section
http://www.naph.org/template.cfm?Section=Issues_Advocacy

The National Association of Public Hospitals and Health Systems (Issues Advocacy section) Web pages present the position of major hospitals and healthcare systems on major healthcare policy issues. It is a good site for the hospital perspective on current health reform issues.

National Coalition on Healthcare
http://www.nchc.org/

Its Web site contains a section called "Did You Know," which briefly reviews key issues in health reform, and a section titled "Policy Studies," which contains more in-depth analysis of these issues.

National Health Policy Forum
http://www.nhpf.org

The Web site provides summaries of and links to reports from sessions between government staff and experts from many healthcare settings.

Stateline.org
http://www.stateline.org

Stateline.org was founded in order to help journalists, policy makers, and engaged citizens become better informed about innovative public policies. The organization's Web site is operated by the Pew Center on the States, a research organization administered by the University of Richmond, and funded by the Pew Charitable Trusts. Its Healthcare section contains stories and statistics related to healthcare issues and reform.

UCLA Center for Health Policy Research
http://www.healthpolicy.ucla.edu/

The site contains extensive pdf reports, briefs, and data relating to policy issues with a focus on California.

YourDoctorintheFamily.com
http://www.yourdoctorinthefamily.com

YourDoctorintheFamily.com is a Web site set up in January 2002 by a group of physicians who are disaffected with the healthcare system. This group of physicians states that what is "especially intolerable to us is the degree to which the interests of physicians are being *systematically* separated from the interests of their patients. The programmed destruction of the traditional doctor-patient relationship leaves both doctors and patients increasingly isolated and marginalized in a complex and hostile health care system." The organization's Web site presents a somewhat irreverent view of health policy and reform issues from the physician's viewpoint.

Glossary

Access   Ability of persons needing healthcare services to obtain appropriate care in a timely manner. While access is not the same as having health insurance coverage, having such coverage is a major factor in having access to care.

Acute care   Short-term care, often of an intense nature, for injury or illness; can include hospitalization.

AHCPR   Agency for Health Care Policy and Research, now renamed AHRQ. This agency deals with issues of healthcare policy and health services research. (Formerly known as NCHSR, National Center for Health Services Research.)

AHRQ   The Agency for Health Care Research and Quality (formerly AHCPR) deals with issues of healthcare policy, health services research, health quality issues, and health practice guidelines. The agency also conducts several important surveys to obtain data on healthcare expenditures and some hospital-related data.

Ambulatory care   Sometimes also called outpatient care, that is, care given to people in a doctor's office, outpatient center, or other special parts of hospitals, for which patients do not need to stay overnight in any type of formal healthcare facility.

CDC   The Centers for Disease Control and Prevention is the federal agency that includes the National Center for Health Statistics (NCHS) and has responsibility for a variety of prevention-oriented programs, including chronic diseases as well as acute problems and infectious disease.

Chronic disease   Medical conditions that persist over time. Chronic problems may lead to permanent healthcare problems. Chronic care can occur in many settings, such as outpatient, hospital, or long-term care facilities.

245

CMS The Centers for Medicare and Medicaid Services is the new name for the Health Care Financing Administration (HCFA). This is the agency that administers the Medicare and Medicaid programs, as well as the Children's Health Insurance Program (CHIP).

Copayment A portion of the healthcare expenses that the patient must provide. Generally a health insurance plan or health maintenance organization (HMO) will specify this amount to the insured person.

Deductible A portion of healthcare costs that the insured person must pay first before insurance payment begins.

DHHS The Department of Health and Human Services.

DRG Diagnosis-related group. This is the current payment approach used for Medicare hospital payment. Rather than paying for specific services as they occur in the hospital, hospital charges are paid for a bundled group of all services as related to a federally specified list of diagnoses.

Entitlement programs Healthcare programs that certain categories of people are entitled to. For example, most people at sixty-five years of age are entitled to Medicare because of their payroll taxes during the years when they were employed.

Fee-for-service Payment of specific fees (generally to a physician) for each service that a patient receives, such as the office examination, a shot, or a diagnostic test.

Gatekeeper physician Generally a primary care physician who functions as the regular source of care for a patient and who must approve the use of specialists and other services as part of a managed care plan.

GDP Gross domestic product. It is a measure of all the goods and services produced by a nation in a given year.

Generalist A family practice, general internal medicine, or general pediatrics physician. These types of physicians often function as gatekeepers within certain managed care systems.

HCFA The Health Care Financing Administration was the name of the agency that administers the Medicare and Medicaid programs, as well as the Children's Health Insurance Program (CHIP). The agency has now been renamed the Centers for Medicare and Medicaid Services (CMS).

HMO A health maintenance organization is a type of managed care organization that generally provides comprehensive medical care for a set predetermined annual fee per employee, generally with only modest copayments and no deductibles.

Home health services Nursing, special therapy services such as physical therapy, and health-related homemaker services that are provided to patients in their homes, generally because the patients have a chronic illness or a disability that makes them unable to leave their home to receive services.

Hospital services The healthcare services that patients receive while they are overnight patients in a hospital. Similar to inpatient services.

Independent Practice Association (IPA) A legal entity that physicians in private practice join so that the organization can represent them in the negotiation of contracts with managed care organizations.

Infant mortality rate The number of deaths that occur to infants in the first year of life. The infant mortality rate is often considered one of the best indicators of how well a country's healthcare system is working.

Infectious diseases Diseases that are transmitted in various ways, through the air, through water, and through sexual modes of transmission. Currently, many of the most important infectious diseases are sexually transmitted and transmitted through the bloodstream, such as AIDS.

Inpatient services Services received while a patient is temporarily confined to a hospital or nursing home, where he or she stays overnight.

Insurance carrier The insurer.

Insured The person who contracts with an insurance company for coverage; also known as the policy holder or the subscriber.

Long-term care Services received as part of extended care needed for people with chronic illnesses, mental illnesses, or serious disabilities. These services are often provided in nursing homes and often focus on basic daily needs.

Managed care A system of provision and payment for healthcare that unites the functions of health insurance and the actual delivery of care.

MCO A managed care organization.

Medicaid A joint federal-state program that provides health insurance coverage to many of the poor.

Medicare The federal program that provides health insurance coverage to the elderly and to some disabled people.

Medigap Commercial health insurance policies purchased by people with Medicare coverage to cover the expenses (such as drugs) not covered by Medicare; the insurance also provides coverage for certain other costs within Medicare, such as required copayments for certain services.

Morbidity   Sickness.

Mortality   Death.

Neonatal death rate   Refers to deaths of infants in the first twenty-eight days of life. The neonatal death rate is generally considered more sensitive to genetic factors and conditions during the birth, as contrasted to the infant mortality rate.

Organized medicine   Refers to the activities of physicians, generally to protect their own interests, such as organizing and acting through groups such as the American Medical Association (AMA).

Outcome   The results of healthcare delivery, of great interest now as a way to measure the effectiveness of the healthcare delivery system.

Out-of-pocket costs   Costs of healthcare that are paid by the patient, the consumer of services. Depending on the type of health insurance that a person has, this would include required deductibles and copayments for care.

Outpatient services   Healthcare services that are provided that are not part of an overnight stay in a hospital (as contrasted to inpatient services).

Payer   The party that actually makes the payment for services covered by an insurance policy. Generally, the payer is the same as the insurer.

Physician-hospital organization   A legal entity that is formed between a hospital and a physician group, generally to share a market, patients, and other mutual interests.

Preexisting condition   A condition (either physical or mental) that existed prior to the beginning of an insurance policy. Some policies will exclude these kinds of conditions. Generally workplace policies will not.

Preferred provider organization (PPO)   These types of organizations are related to managed care. Often insurance companies set up their own contracts with companies and with providers for the provision of care. In these types of groups, the insurance company makes a contractual arrangement with a group of providers or individual providers for provision of services at a discounted fee.

Premiums   Amount charged by an insurance company for a policy.

Primary care   Medical care provided in the office or clinic by a provider such as a doctor, physician's assistant, or nurse practitioner. This is the first level of contact by a patient within the healthcare delivery system.

Prospective Payment System (PPS) In this type of payment system, how much is to be paid for a particular service is predetermined, as contrasted with retrospective reimbursement.

Reimbursement Amount paid to a provider (i.e., doctor, hospital, etc.) by the insurance company or managed care group. This payment may only be a portion of what the provider charges. In a managed care setting, the amount may have been negotiated in advance.

Resource-based relative value scale (RBRVS) A system in place in Medicare to determine physician fees. Each treatment or visit with a physician is assigned a "relative value" based on the training, skill, and time that is required to treat the condition.

Retrospective reimbursement The amount to be paid is determined on the basis of the actual costs incurred, generally after services have been delivered.

Safety net Programs that enable people to receive healthcare services (as well as many other social services) even if they lack the resources to pay for those services. Medicaid is an example of a safety net program in healthcare, as are community health centers. These are generally government programs.

Single-payer system A proposal for healthcare reform that emphasizes the creation of a single organization, typically a government agency, to pay all healthcare claims.

Uncompensated care Services provided to consumers as a charity without the person paying for the services.

Welfare programs Means-tested programs that provide income or services to people with low enough incomes to qualify for the program. In healthcare, Medicaid is an example of a welfare program.

Index

About the Authors

Jennie Jacobs Kronenfeld is professor of sociology at Arizona State University. She has published over 100 articles on medical sociology, public health, and health care policy. She has authored, coauthored, or edited over 20 books on a wide variety of topics related to health and social policy, professional development, health policy concerns, and research in sociology of health care.

Michael R. Kronenfeld is director of the Educational Resources Center at the A.T. Still University of the Health Sciences, Mesa Arizona. He has published over 20 articles. In 2001 he received the Ida and George Eliot Prize from the Medical Library Association for the publication that was most effective in furthering medical librarianship in 2001. In 2003 he received the David A. Kronick Traveling Fellowship, also from the Medical Library Association, for research on trends and future directions for academic medical libraries.